HEALING
THROUGH
WISDOM

YOUR ESSENTIAL GUIDE TO LIVING WELL

CHRISSY HELMER

Printed in the United States of America

ISBN: 978-1-09-157404-5

Eco Chic Life Inc.
1661 East Monte Vista Avenue
Suite Q102
Vacaville, CA 95688
(707) 624-6168
www.ecochiclife.net/htwbook

Follow @chrissyhelmer @ecochiclife

Cover Design: Jen Ybarra
Editor: Marcy McCoy

This book was proudly printed on recycled,
acid-free paper with chlorine-free ink.

A percent of sales from this book go to:
Children's Health Defense
www.childrenshealthdefense.org
We Love Our City
www.weloveourcity.org

For everyone on a journey to heal themselves and the world

CONTENTS

ENDORSEMENTS

"Wisdom is something we all need in this day and age. In the Bible, King Solomon asked for wisdom above all else. In a world full of information, it can get pretty confusing at times. It is refreshing to find a good source of knowledge on a number of topics on healthy living. *Healing Through Wisdom* is such a book. Chrissy covers many topics, and I believe you will find the wisdom and knowledge to make those decisions for a healthy lifestyle for yourself and those you love."

Beni Johnson — Senior Pastor of Bethel Church;
Author of *Healthy and Free*

"I have known Chrissy Helmer for nearly twenty years, and I have watched her journey of faith and healing. *Healing Through Wisdom* is far more than healthy living ideas and one more holistic offering for the bookshelves. This book is a collection of wisdom and insight, gleaned from her life lived helping others, and her journey of success in the areas of health, healing, wholeness, and the joy of living your best life. I would highly recommend the content and the coaching within

9

these pages, but more than that, I would recommend Chrissy and her unique perspective and expertise in these time-tested practices of living whole in spirit, soul, and body."

Dave Patterson — Lead Pastor of The Father's House

"This book is a must-read for all who are interested in living a fulfilled life of health and empowerment. Chrissy does an amazing job of explaining the value and the 'why' for choosing a lifestyle of health and complete wellness. She covers all the areas that make a well-rounded, balanced, healthy life. She includes all four aspects of physical, emotional, mental, and spiritual health. The beautiful part about Chrissy is that she lives this life fully and completely, and is always growing and learning. She also inspires everyone around her to want to embrace this amazing lifestyle. She is a walking book of knowledge and practicum, and makes it so easy and simple that you know you can do it. In person, just like in this beautiful book, she is always there to help, inspire, guide, and teach you the best way to live a fulfilled life. She is an exhilarating, dynamo speaker who leaves you motivated to be the you that was created to soar. I encourage everyone to have this book in their personal library. It will keep you energized to continue this wonderful journey of life."

Gayle Belanger — Author;
Founder and Director of Live Free Ministry

"As you begin to read this book, it doesn't take long to realize that Chrissy is not only passionate, but a forerunner in the area of healing and wholeness. She is recognized in our community for being a strong, leading voice which many have gone to for help. I have personally benefited from her knowledge and expertise during a challenging season of my life. This book does an excellent job building a bridge between the 'average Joe' and the self-proclaimed 'health gurus' out there. Thank you, Chrissy, for writing *Healing Through Wisdom* and helping us on our journey to a happier, healthier life!"

Shane Guy — Pastor and School Director

"Taboo topics are brought to light, unraveled, backed by research, and supported with alternative methods. Chrissy is a wellspring of knowledge in healthy minds, bodies, and spirits. This book is a gamer changer for today!"

Nicole Van Staden — Former Educator

"Chrissy has a heart for people and a heart for teaching, and it really shows in this book, *Healing Through Wisdom*. Her real life, raw approach, along with current research concerning our everyday health, diet, and hygiene decisions are insightful and useful. To God be the glory for the truth being exposed, and for getting our bodies back into balance."

**Claudette Coughenour — Midwife;
Founder of New Life Birthing Services**

"I have been friends with Chrissy for nineteen years. I watched her get married, become a mother of three, work hard to become a business owner, blossom into a knowledgeable health advocate, teacher, speaker, coach, mentor, sports mom, city leader, spokesperson, and now an author. Her passion and tireless tenacity for greater knowledge and understanding in everything she is involved with is inspiring, and so many of us benefit from it. Thank you for working hard and 'going after it' so we can live better lives. Your love for God, people, and truth is evident in who you are and all you do! Thank you, Chrissy!"

Tammy Hawkins — Pastor and Author

"*Healing Through Wisdom* is not your typical book. It is a reference that you will continue to go back to in order to find the answers you have been searching for. Chrissy is not only my friend, but someone who has paved the way regarding truth, health, and healing through holistic health practices in her personal journey and as a business owner. Her mission is her life, and her life is her mission.

As someone who has battled cancer, given only a year to live, and has overcome it by natural means in just ninety days, I know firsthand how important it is to have our spiritual, mental, and physical health be in complete alignment with one another. Our bodies were meant to heal fully, but we need to remove the interference. Chrissy's book gives you powerful insight on how to be your own best advocate when it comes to your health and wellness. She has such a passion and a desire to see families, communities, and nations changed and shaped in a way that brings healing and wholeness to all."

Andrea Thompson — Health Coach and Advocate;
Author of *I Am Resilient*

"We have had the pleasure and blessing of knowing Chrissy Helmer on a personal level for over a decade. She is a person who is passionate about everything she does, and this book is no exception to that. The information contained in *Healing Through Wisdom* is a shining example of Chrissy's passion and desire to share her knowledge and personal experience with the world. Not only are the chapters in this book packed with tons of information about achieving complete and total health, but they read as if she is sitting right in front of you. With a no holds barred approach, Chrissy's personal experience, humor, encouragement, and the wisdom found within these pages help to deliver a powerful tool for you to utilize in order to bring your physical, mental, and spiritual health to an optimal level!"

Dr. David and Teresa Conner — Chiropractor;
Owners of Conner Chiropractic Care Corp.;
General Manager of Maximum Fitness, LLC

INTRODUCTION

HEART FOR HEALTH

WHOLENESS (MIND, BODY, AND SPIRIT)

Healing Through Wisdom is my heart for wholeness for every person to live well, love well, and be well. I have been in the health world since I had my first son, Gabe, in 2001. He had some health complications which led me to do my own research. Ultimately, that pointed me down a holistic path which I am very grateful for.

I have been a holistic health educator and a doula since 2007. Through being a doula, I've had the pleasure of working with the most incredible midwives and holistic practitioners. When I was studying to become a doula and an educator, I was honored and privileged to work for a chiropractor, which ultimately helped affirm my holistic path.

Since 2011, I have owned a holistic, sustainable, organic, give-back brick and mortar boutique: Eco Chic. I have poured my blood, sweat, and tears into educating people about their diet, their mindsets, and the products they use in their homes, on their bodies, and beyond. I have also been the host of a podcast since 2017, addressing these topics and helping people take their lives to the next level.

I have always been a huge advocate for mental and spiritual health. I genuinely believe that wholeness needs to incorporate mind, body, and spirit. As someone who grew up in church, Christian schools, ministry, and the nonprofit world, I have a burning desire that believers, and those who are on incredible missions with purpose, would not neglect their physical health any longer. What I'm about to say may come off a bit intense, but I believe we would have many people still on this side of heaven with us had they known this powerful information about healing their bodies through wisdom.

The heart behind this book is not only to educate, empower, and inspire people to live whole, healthy, powerful, strong, and long lives, but that we would take this message to every person in our sphere. My heart is that we will see disease and pain decrease and that we will see the dependency on our medical system, Big Pharma, and toxic foods not only exposed but changed.

KNOWLEDGE IS POWER

"It doesn't matter how many people don't get it.
It matters how many people do."
— Vani Hari

You will hear me say this throughout the book, and it's because I truly believe it: when we know better, we do better. I don't think people who choose toxic products are consciously or knowingly harming themselves. On the other hand, we have so much information from YouTube, social media, audiobooks, and podcasts that it's almost hard not to know the truth about what's going on within our food and medical industries.

Since owning a holistic-minded store, I have seen an enormous shift in the last few years in people's consciousness, mindset, awareness, and energy toward wellness. The first few years we were open, we were certainly mocked and made fun of because people did not understand basic holistic remedies, like essential oils or echinacea, which are now very common. I am thankful for the mediums that are getting the word out about health and wellness.

We still have a lot of work to do because all the information available can be overwhelming at times, especially when it comes to *What should I actually eat?* or *What vitamins should I actually take?* We have a surplus of information at our disposal, which can lead some people to not make a decision based on their overwhelmed state. On the flip side, some people are of the mindset that they know the truth about the harmful products and what they can do to their health or their home, yet they choose to ignore it and have a "whatever" mindset.

Our egos, unresolved pains, wounds, and issues will sabotage us from living well mentally, spiritually, physically, and emotionally. The sad part is it doesn't have to be this way. That is why a portion of this book focuses on mindsets and emotional health because it plays a much more significant role in our physical health than we typically give credit.

So often the fitness industry is focused just on the body and working out—and there's a place and a time for that. Physical fitness does matter; however, we can't neglect what we're putting in our bodies, what we're saying, what we're thinking about, what we're meditating on, and what we're affirming. We also can't just eat organic, paleo, keto, Whole30, "clean," or whatever is working for you—which is very important and does affect every aspect of our health, including our energy and sleep. But again, we can't ignore what's going on in our heart or overlook the importance of fitness. It's actually said that health is 80 percent what you eat, the products you use, and what you think, and 20 percent physical fitness.

I'm sure a yoga or kickboxing instructor is reading this right now and wants to throw down with me. Again, being physically fit matters! Even if it's just walking thirty minutes a day, or a five- to ten-minute HIIT workout. Studies show there is tremendous value in how physical activity affects our health. I believe working out helps in many different areas, and I do not take away from it at all. I work out at least three days a week, myself. The point here is that we cannot focus solely on diet or emotional health or physical health; we need to bring balance to each of these areas to be truly whole.

Growing up as a believer, I have seen and fully believe in miracles, and I love the supernatural. I also love Bethel Church and their team, and I regularly attend a spirit-filled church. I want to be so clear in sharing this: I love God, I love the Church, and I love prayer. Prayer is a blessing; it has its place, it is amazing, and I'm thankful for it. The supernatural and signs and wonders are one hundred percent for today. Sometimes miracles come in ways we don't expect, like a book, a holistic boutique, a health coach, a dream, a divine connection, or through wisdom. Let's not put limits on how the healing will come, but, instead, let's be open to all that is possible as we journey through this book together.

DISCLAIMER

I have written this book from my heart, my experience, and my interactions with friends, clients, and customers over the last twelve years. This book is much more than stats, articles, research, podcasts, and hundreds of hours down a rabbit hole of truth; it's real people in my life and my store daily.

This book is a little unconventional in a few ways, as it has been written from carpool lines, football games, and from the family room while asking kids to *please keep it down for the tenth time*. It would have been easy to make this a safe and pretty book with remedies for your headaches, eczema, and cough. It would be easy to keep certain things to myself or in a safe bubble, but change will never happen if I keep these truths tucked away. I would be robbing you and future generations from divine health, change, and awakening. This book will be here long after me, and I consider this book a complete game changer.

If you don't know me, I'd like to shine some light on my personality. As a child, I wanted to be the president, a doctor, and a teacher. I am a born-cheerleader. I went to a school that had a focus on faith, character, performing arts, and community involvement. Growing up, I got in trouble for talking too much— they had "talking tallies" in my classroom, and I got one every day.

I was raised in a culture of empowerment, faith, "go get 'em," and was taught anything is possible. My family often called my uncle and me "the mayor!" My dad is one of the most fearless people I know, and he and my mom taught me to confront anyone and anything at any cost.

I am a Di on the DISC personality test, and a strong Eight with a Seven wing on the Enneagram. I am very convicted about the things in this book, and I operate with high energy (some call it hyper). I am driven, motivated, and passionate, yet I love to have fun, joke around, and be completely real. There is a lot of sarcasm and urban lingo weaved throughout this book that I hope you pick up on. You have permission to laugh at my jokes, feel the passion and love coming from every word, enjoy this book fully, and feel like it's just you and me talking. My love language is words, so hearing all your encouraging messages, posts, notes, and reviews will be my oxygen.

As you read on, I want you to know that you don't have to think like me, vote like me, believe like me, pray like me, eat like me, or live like me. I only ask that you read it from your highest self, not your conditioned self. We don't need to share the same beliefs or convictions to not only respect and honor each other, but to be in community. No matter where you stand, please know I stand with you for your best health, your inner greatness, and your best life. Feel free to toss any part of this book out that isn't for you, but don't let that keep you from the gold that *is* for you.

This book may bring up things that question your trust and security in many beliefs or systems. It also might awaken and enlighten you to things you didn't know. It might be the very key you needed for your breakthrough. It might stir something in you to reform a system; I pray it does. It might be the flame that consumes a movement of people to overhaul corruption and compromise and see better for ourselves, our communities, our futures, our children, and our earth.

I am strongly convicted to share what I know, even when it comes at a cost, especially in the time we live in where what's popular typically is what's politically correct, or—better yet— what doesn't touch anything of meaning at all. So many people are afraid to take a stand for what they believe in or even share their own stories or experiences.

I hope this book will give many people courage not just to share, but to take action to change, reform, speak up, and stand up. I also ask you to stand up for me, my business, and this movement as we could call this piece of work counter-cultural. I declare that fear can go to hell. Peaceful warriors are rising, and we won't remain silent.

Please read with caution, without distraction, assumption, judgment, or bias if you want to extract every piece of wisdom and truth. I encourage you to read this book with a deep conviction to empower, equip, and inspire people to understand the great importance of health and how it's connected to your purpose, impact, and future. I believe wisdom comes to us when we are ready.

As I have discovered through the last twelve years, we continually see new information released, and anything on health is not concrete. I do believe there are some core principles we should abide by and as we grow. We should be increasing our faith, our stewardship, and our diligence with our health, our time, our passions, our relationships, and our resources.

I want to make it clear that the views and opinions in this book may not be the views of my church, family, vendors, friends, or network. What I have written is not about right or wrong, left or right, or taking sides; it's about gaining insight that cannot only change your life but history—especially in America.

For my friends in the health industry that live this, and for my friends who have healed from chronic illness and already live non-toxic, you may find there will be shocking new sources of information not found packaged in this way before. I can't wait to hear not only what has impacted you, but how you have applied what's inside of this book and seen a turnaround in your mind, body, and spirit.

To be very clear in this disclaimer: I am not anti-government, anti-medical system, or anti-vaccines, but I am very anti-corruption, anti-deception, anti-harmful agendas, anti-population control, and anti-toxic chemicals. We should have access to affordable and accessible alternative healthcare options, and our personal care, home environment, food, products, and medications should not be harming us. Companies that do harm should be held liable and responsible for these damages and deceptions. I care far too much about my family, friends, future, community, planet, and the wellbeing of humanity to ignore the current conditions.

People say friends don't let friends drive drunk. I say friends don't let friends shop at chain stores. Friends don't let friends put cancer-causing chemicals on their bodies, in their bodies, or in their homes. Friends don't let friends keep making poor, harmful choices when they have the answers and resources for them.

I completely respect and understand everybody is on their

journey and everybody is ready for different things at different times. I think there is an honorable and respectful way to share information like this with your friends, families, and coworkers without coming off like an annoying, crazy, holistic health nut. I will be sharing about how to approach friends and family throughout this book, full of honest, sacred stories, information, insights, and resources. You may already know what we are up against in our health and food systems, yet I know there is still gold in here for you. There indeed is something for everyone. I have yet to find a resource like this that has weaved as much information, facts, humor, and application in a multi-dimensional approach—hence why I wrote this book!

I'm sharing this with you because I care, and because I believe we are better than our current state of health. I'm sharing because I want you to be empowered, informed, inspired, and educated at a whole new level. There may be parts of this book you already know, and there may be some parts that are brand new to you. There may be one key in here for you, or there may be five keys in here for you. This ultimately may be a message you feel called to share with your community.

What I don't want you to do with this book is to just read it and then not apply it or share it. This book is a mission, and I am asking you to accept this call and join me on a journey to creating the healthiest communities possible. Join me in raising awareness, speaking the truth, and creating lasting change.

> *"In a gentle way, you can shake the world."*
> *— Gandhi*

CHAPTER ONE
FROM LUCKY CHARMS TO LEMON WATER

MY HOLISTIC SALVATION

I want to get some things out of the way before we dive into my Lucky Charms childhood:

1. I don't live in a tiny house.
2. I don't own a Prius.
3. I don't live in a yurt.
4. I don't wear exclusively hemp clothing.
5. I don't smell like patchouli.

Now that we have cleared that up! People often think my parents must be health gurus, and I grew up on a compound garden from the time I could walk. Yeah, no. Let me be clear: *that is the furthest thing from the truth.* For starters, I was born to teenage parents in the eighties—an era where people didn't question or research things or even have what we have today. There was no technology to get that type of information quickly, let alone on your own. Lord, when I had my first son I had to go to the library, for the love, to get books on health!

The generation before my parents actually enjoyed raw milk and organic food. Co-ops were popular, and there were not a lot of systems, medications, or the epidemics we see now. Yeah, they might have smoked in cars, but they were not as medicated as we are now.

I wasn't breastfed, I got mercury fillings, ate junk food, and I was vaccinated. (I'm still getting over that.) I grew up on Lucky Charms, Fruity Pebbles, Coke, and Little Debbie, y'all! When something was wrong, we went to the doctor, and we probably used antibiotics too much. We didn't question the system or know any better, because I truly believe when we know better, we do better.

Sadly, even though both of my parents are young, they suffer from many different things due to lifestyle, childhood, medications, diet, and life. They are still working, enjoying life, golfing, shopping, up and around, and all that good stuff, but definitely not at optimal health and energy. My grandma is seventy-five and going strong, but still has some health challenges. My other grandma is still working at the age of seventy-nine. My grandpa died of cancer in his fifties, and my other grandpa hasn't been well for at least ten years. It also saddens me to say I had an uncle die at twenty-two from cancer. On top of all that, mental health issues run rampant in my family, and digestive and hormone issues are common.

Thankfully, my parents have invested in making changes, getting more information, taking baby steps, and they are on a path of healing. They are involved in our kids' lives, supporters of everything I do, and great examples. They only did what they knew at the time, as most of us do. Many of us have been victims of the system offering us only pills and procedures that leave us with other issues to resolve. Getting to the root of it has never been the agenda in modern medicine. Reading labels wasn't a discussion in the eighties. Questioning your provider, being your own advocate, and "going back to nature" wasn't common even a decade ago.

I am the only woman in my family who isn't on thyroid medication, or any other medicine to be transparent. According to Dr. John Bergman, 60 percent of Americans are on prescription medications. This epidemic is contributing to our declining health crisis. Y'all. I should have written a chapter on this alone. Lord, help us.

I believe parents do the best they can with what they have and what they know at the time. I am deeply thankful that my parents were fun, caring, kind, loving, faith-filled, and raised me well—despite feeding me Hamburger Helper and Cup O'Noodles for dinner. I will give it to my mom though, she gave us Flintstones Vitamins as kids. (Which I now know were just crunchy clusters of sugar, wheat, corn, and crap.) She also cooked, but nothing was organic, and we ate a lot of sugar. Shout-out to the bubble gum antibiotic bottle that was like a household staple in the fridge! *Mom, I know you're laughing with me.*

As a teenager, I was addicted to fast food. I ate it almost every day, and got strep throat at least once a year. I loved Doritos and Coca-Cola. I slathered myself in toxic, hormone-disrupting Bath and Body Works lotions, and sprayed my curly hair with cancer-causing hairsprays (shout-out to Aussie Sprunch Spray in the purple bottle, circa 1996). Shocking, right?

From the age of eighteen to twenty-two, I thought a good breakfast was a warm, morning bun and frap from Starbucks. I didn't know better. I was addicted to sugar. I truly didn't realize what I consumed was directly connected to my headaches, fevers, and roller coaster of emotions—or that I had celiac, a corn allergy, and a gene mutation. I was a hot mess most of the time, but from the outside, I looked healthy because I was "skinny," athletic, and had great skin (thanks, Grandma). I was also nineteen, so there's that.

Before I knew better, I would burn toxic, chemical candles

(yes, even soy is garbage) and wonder why everybody had a cough. I washed our clothes in hormone-disrupting, sinus-bothering, headache-triggering, skin-irritating detergents. You know, the ones that have bright colors and are in all the commercials?

Honestly, I would probably be very unhealthy today if it wasn't for all the research I did and the changes I made starting at the age of twenty and heavily at the age of twenty-seven. My healing and detoxing journey is still in motion.

Speaking of unhealthy, can we address that? Usually when we hear "unhealthy," we think fat, bad skin, someone on meds, lazy, and the list goes on. There are people who *look* very healthy who are not. Beneath it all, their gallbladder and liver are dying, they have leaky gut, and their reproductive system is under attack. Their mitochondria are way off (I felt very smart using that word until I had to spell check it), and their energy levels, immune system, and sleep are all jacked. Healthy is not a *look*.

I am thankful I wasn't on the verge of dying or suffering from a disease. I was simply a product of the system. I was one of the sheep, and I was pretty asleep to the truth. I was a victim of propaganda where I accepted and believed *this isn't bad for me.* Not to mention, I was a hardcore athlete, playing high school softball, volleyball, and travel ball. Thankfully, my natural personality is high energy and hyper (with the perfect dose of ADD), or I don't think I could have performed at the level that I did. I'm sharing this with you because if anybody thinks they can't do this, take a look at my story and *know* it is possible.

BE A CHANGE AGENT

My next confession, since it's just you and me, is probably the part I have the most guilt and shame about. Don't worry, I have the tools to heal—I've handled it. I'm good, really! I would reward my toddlers with McDonald's Happy Meals and meet friends for our Friday playdate at the McDonald's PlayPlace while we all enjoyed our six-piece nugget meal. Yes, you should read that again to make sure that's what I said. And we wondered why our kids were so out of control, and had digestive issues, eczema, and frequent chronic colds! Let's not get started with my oldest son's one-of-a-kind asthma that caused him to throw up at least four days a week. Hear me, I don't think a six-piece nugget meal is going to do all that, but you get the point.

Speaking of that, my oldest son was vaccine-injured, and we found out he had a gene mutation, sensitivities, and much more. There is a lot to share on that, but for privacy and page sake, I'll keep it short. He had been "sick" from birth, and almost died. He went from one doctor to the next, despite being exclusively breastfed. I took him in for a checkup because I knew something wasn't right. When they checked his oxygen levels, the doctor freaked, alarms went off, and they said, "Your son could die if he doesn't get support right now. He has to get to the hospital in Sacramento." Mind you, I'm twenty years old. I am on my way out of town, and my husband works an hour and a half away. *Scary!*

That next week was horrible. Staying in the hospital is the worst on its own. Add in judgmental, rude nurses, and test after test, after test, after test, after test, after test (yeah, that many) for them to "not be sure." One day to the next was hard. They treated and tested him for numerous things and finally released us, deciding it wasn't on a list of specific diagnoses, and it was some infection or bacteria or something. Over the next year, he continued to get sick. RSV. Heart murmur. Speech delay. Infections. All of this led me to go full-on mama bear and figure out *what the actual.*

I would say my experience with all of this, along with my health stuff and birth experiences (one natural epidural, one semi-natural, and one home-birth), being a health educator, being at births, and working with families gave me a passion for helping, educating, and empowering people. As I mentioned earlier, I wanted to be a doctor and a teacher when I grew up. I can proudly say that's pretty much what I get to do (in a holistic sense) for myself and my community. My findings didn't come overnight though.

I am so thankful I had one family friend who was like an aunt to me. She was my doula at two of my births, and she mentioned several books, herbs, and ideas to me before it was a thing. That alone opened up a road for me to alternatives and wisdom. The journey was long, and the fight was hard. I was doing all this in the 2001-2010 timeframe when hardly anyone had a doula, used essential oils, and read up on autism, vaccines, or allergies. I felt alone and afraid a lot of the time, not to mention *crazy*.

Thankfully, I had one other friend who was a young mom and had something similar happen to her daughter. The doctors said her daughter had autism and would never X-Y-Z. Let me happily tell you that after her detox, prayers, wisdom, alternative road, and different choices, this girl is now a 4.0 student, a leader, and she's thriving!

I realize this is not the case for many though. To you, I say *keep fighting*.

I highly recommend reading Dr. Jordan Rubin's story. He was one of my introductions to the truth about this whole holistic world, and he's one of my favorite influences in this arena. His book, *The Maker's Diet*, was my first go-to about all things health. Dr. Rubin is also the founder of Garden of Life, a brand that was established in 1988 and one I've been using since 2004. Dr. Joseph Mercola was my other go-to, long before Pinterest or social media was even a thing. He is the OG, for sure. Thankfully, there are many fantastic, legit resources out there, along with technology to help educate and empower you quickly. Be careful though. There are a lot of fake, shallow, and not-so-good ones out there, too. Choose wisely. You can check the Reference section in the back for my trusted ones.

> **"When you remain in peace,**
> **you remain in power."**
> — *Joel Osteen*

Without going into a full-on vaccine education section and laying out all the ingredients yet (I'll do that in *Enemies of Health*), I do need to share this part of my journey with you, as it is a huge part. I am so thankful for doctors, like Dr. Sears and Dr. Tenpenny, and documentaries, like *The Greater Good, Trace Amounts, Vaxxed: From Cover-Up to Catastrophe*, and *Stink!* that I've learned so much from about this topic.

Dealing with food sensitivities, allergies, gene mutations, heart murmurs, and reactions is not a joke. I think I slept three hours a night for three to four years straight. That season was tough, to say the least. It wasn't happening to me though; it was happening *for* and through me.

I would not be writing this book if I had not experienced all of that. It led me to educate myself, which then led me to want to share what I knew with those who are ready. (Note the difference between sharing with those we are ready and with everyone. Major key.)

Any mother who loves her child will do *anything* to ensure they are healthy, well, and going to live their best life. The funny thing is, along our journey, we were told my son would not be able to do many things. Thanks to wisdom, prayer, discipline, application, alternative health, and support, my son is a top athlete, business owner, a fantastic student, and is a strong leader. We deal with flares of things from time to time (mostly due to food choices), and I'd love to have him do an annual detox—which he would benefit from greatly—but he is a teenager. He gets to choose. (Certain things anyway.) All I know is that I'm praying for his future wife. She will need to be strong, outspoken, holistic, and on it. The things we teach, instill, and impart to our kids—be it faith, health, leadership, finances—are as much for now as they are for their adult life.

"You can fuel your body and
wellness, or you can fuel disease."

Did you know most people have either a sensitivity, intolerance, allergy, or deficiency of some kind? It doesn't always show up as a hospital visit or disease, but it's there, and unfortunately, it will manifest in one way or another some day. Pending your upbringing, environment, choices, overall health (mind, body, spirit), microbiome, hormones, history, blood type, and genome, one day some part of you will say *I'm done!* Then you will be on a time crunch to detox, learn, heal, and change all at once. All of that can and will work, but wouldn't you rather prevent?

When anyone comes to me with some ailment, pain, or issue, they say, *"Tell me what to do or what I need,"* because no one wants to be struggling, sick, tired, or stressed. Our hearts were made to be whole, our lives were made to be full, and our bodies were made to be strong. That is the original design. Our bodies carry frequencies and light. Our bodies are capable and for us. We need to help them, not hurt them. Your body will only be able to take all those chemicals and abuse for so long. For some, their bodies may not take it for very long. It might be anxiety, psoriasis, digestive issues, headaches, full-blown MS, or cancer. I don't know. But I do know there is a better way. Let's be on the offense and prevent with wisdom. When you know better, you do better.

I share all of this because I would never want you to think that this journey has just been so simple and easy for me. I mentioned my first son, but my middle son went through horrible eczema due to an omega deficiency, chemical allergies, and a gluten allergy. Same with my daughter. I was given RhoGAM shots with my first two pregnancies. I was also "forced" to have a nasal flu shot when I was pregnant. (I was told it didn't have any metals in it.) Within weeks of having my middle son, we both got strep. Imagine having strep with a newborn and a toddler. It was awful.

I'm not sharing every story or sickness, but I want to give you a glimpse. Childhood infections are connected to our mental health. Dr. Ben Lynch has fantastic information on this. My middle son also had dental work done when he was four-years-old that I *deeply* regret (heavy metal city). It gave him metal toxicity, which ultimately affects the way he processes. I can't believe I let a dentist bully me into a decision that I fought and shared concerns on (mind you, I was twenty-six). He made me feel like a horrible mother, uneducated, and crazy for wanting to go another route.

I know many people have children with allergies, delays, and disabilities. I truly understand. I've dealt with therapies, 504s, IEPS, and meeting after meeting. Horrific days and good days. All of it is still pretty real and raw, and my teens aren't ready for me to share in depth. I am thankful for what they have given me the green light to share, and I know I would not be the woman I am today if it wasn't for being their mom. I am thankful I have three strong kids, as it has taught me, broke me, healed me, and made me a professional researcher and advocate of health.

> *"What you eat, think, feel, are exposed to, and do every day is far more important than your genetics. Your health destiny is not fated, it is created."*
> — Dr. Jess

BEYOND ORGANIC

Back to me, who I have full permission to share about. One of the hardest parts of my journey was giving up gluten. Giving up the toxic, personal care was no big deal, and organic was the easy part.

At the beginning of my journey, I was more focused on organic than organic and nutrient-dense. I am so thankful for our local Weston A. Price Foundation (you can find a local chapter near you or online), as I was able to learn so much about the power of fermented and living foods. I learned to ask, "*Is this fuel or food?*" and all about eating, shopping, thinking, and choosing mindfully.

I think one of the main reasons giving up gluten was a challenge was that nothing compared to a warm, soft cinnamon roll or French bread. Also, honest confession about me, I would make decisions to give into the cinnamon roll temptation out of comfort, not even hunger. Or even just out of habit. I used to make those choices mindlessly. Now, I make mindful decisions about what I'm eating and even when I'm eating. I make conscious choices to savor, be grateful, and be present. I call it *conscious eating*.

I am incredibly thankful I gave up gluten before I knew I had celiac though. Did you know in America we have seen a 400 percent increase in celiac disease in the last few years alone? There are a few reasons: gene mutations, glyphosate, leaky gut, and many of the enemies I will list in *Enemies of Health*. I'm so grateful I was already on a path of preventative care, a sustainable lifestyle of non-toxic living, and feeling pretty good. It took a naturopath, midwife, and holistic practitioner to get me the right tests and answers. I am sure the mainstream way would have kept throwing creams and pills my way, and I would not be living the life I am today.

> **A lot of people are in a health crisis when they find out or try things differently. The person that comes to mind on this for me is Danielle Walker. She was practically dying and hopeless before she turned to the belief that "food is medicine." If she didn't have the journey she went through, she would not be changing all these lives and writing her amazing cookbooks.**

In 2015 and 2016, I had the worst health years of my life, aside from my vaccine reaction at age one. I was living organic and non-toxic, but I still had organic gluten from time to time (at that time, I made the switch to sprouted and spelt which are low-gluten), but I had yet to find out I had celiac. I thought I had a gluten intolerance or sensitivity (along with 99 percent of America).

I also found out I wasn't taking things for stress like ashwagandha, B-complex, methyl B12, NAC, and holy basil. Between missing out on those great supports with three kids, a business, teaching, leading, and life, I was fighting off one thing after another from November through March (a lot of people need the extra support that time of year). I also wasn't meditating daily or practicing consistent self-compassion.

Those months began with a staph infection on my leg which started as a little cut from diving for a ball on the volleyball court. It was *the worst*. I lost sleep, and I had to do special bandages; my whole body was affected by this infection. I will share that I successfully healed it holistically. But that doesn't mean it was fun. Once the staph infection healed, I got the cough of 2016, and it left me with a dislocated rib. I couldn't laugh or cough without terrible pain. Where was the CBD when I needed it then?

Following that, I got strep, came down with tonsillitis, and lost hearing in one of my ears for over a month. For almost four weeks, I dealt with clogged ears and it was driving me literally *insane*. Hearing yourself talk like you're underwater is maddening. I was doing *all the things*. I finally went to an ENT doctor to see if there was something I was missing. He told me I should get tubes in my ears and start on antibiotics. Thanks, but *no thanks*. I already had tubes as a child, and studies show that it causes scar tissue, hearing issues, lowered immune system, issues in the eustachian tubes, and more. I already have the worst time flying (horrible pain and clogging every time I travel), and I can't scuba dive or drive up to the mountains without a whole healthy ear ritual.

Because of this, I dug even deeper into my health and finally got tested for a *lot of things*—one of them being celiac. I found out everything about my body looked amazing, except I had the HLA-DQ8 gene (celiac). *Seriously.* My naturopath was wise enough to get me on NAC and other stress and immune supports which helped ongoing, and I went one hundred percent gluten- and grain-free. Many don't realize corn, other grains, and even foods like white potatoes can act similarly in the body of someone who has celiac. Although the industry touts corn as a health food, just like gluten, it can cause a leaky gut. This is because, for many people's bodies, the protein in corn can look like gluten, and they "cross-react" to it.

Now, you would think just not eating corn would be enough, but *y'all, it's in everything!* It's even in a lot of organic and gluten-free foods! Most processed foods will, more often than not, reveal some obvious sources of corn, such as high-fructose corn syrup (HFCS), corn oil, and corn starch. But just as gluten sometimes hides under ingredients like MSG and malt, corn can be lurking behind other names (dextrose, xanthan gum, natural flavors, free-flowing agents, vitamin E, ascorbic acid, citric acid, and cellulose).

Also, how about those organic eggs and grass-fed meats you buy? *Corn.* Unless the eggs are pasture-raised (and soy- and corn-free), and the meat is grass-fed and -finished (otherwise it's grain-finished), you have just been duped. I know, right? Corn is also used in the lining of most plastic containers and cups, too. The biggest issue with corn is that 80 percent of it is GMO, so corn is something you want to avoid at all costs.

I know you're thinking, *Chrissy, I live for chips and salsa. I can no longer read your book.* Do not panic! I got you, and I, too, live for chips and queso (cashew-based), chips and guac, and chips and salsa. I found a brand that solved all of this for me, and I will praise Siete brand forever and always, amen. Crisis averted. Five-star book review written. Thank you and amen.

MAKING THE TRANSITION WITH FAMILY

*"You cannot force someone to comprehend
a message that they are not ready to receive.
Still, you must never underestimate
the power of planting a seed."*

Another part of this journey that I get asked a lot about is how I deal with family members who are not on board. I also get asked if my husband and kids are "like me." Of course, with their permission, I will share a little about that here.

It's no secret that my husband is amazing. He's an incredible man who (to name a few things) kills it at fatherhood, does dishes, grocery shops, does the laundry, and supports everything I do, including writing this book and opening and running a store. It's also no secret that he is incredibly stubborn. It's important to note that sharing about holistic health and wellness isn't his calling. It's mine. Getting him on board with everything was definitely a long process. And honestly, it still can be a point of tension for us, especially when it comes to gluten in the house, considering I have celiac. There have been times people have used my spatula or my side of the toaster. There have also been times where he has totally fallen for a greenwashed company and forgot to check the ingredients. We have kids with gluten allergies or gluten sensitivities, too (news flash: that's most people), but they don't care enough yet to go entirely gluten-free.

He is also, like many dads, the fun one. So yes, the kids get special treats with him that they would not get with me. Don't get me wrong, he is woke. He is organic and all of that, but not as extreme as me. I am the mom who offers my kids to trade in the crap for the better, cleaner version. Sometimes I even outright pay my kids for the toxic stuff they get at church, school, and sports so I can dump it in the trash. Thankfully, my kids don't eat fast food (minus Chipotle and whatever they occasionally get with Grandma), and they are good with that. They actually know what good, real food tastes like and enjoy going to high-quality, organic, farm-to-table restaurants with us. They also learn the hard way when they eat things they're not used to; they definitely can struggle with headaches, stomachaches, or come down with a cold within a week of an unhealthy binge (like Christmastime). And when they do, they know who to go to for all the fast remedies.

My oldest son is a hardcore athlete. Performance, growth, and strength connect directly to lifestyle. Look at Michael Phelps, Tom Brady, and the others who are organic. I listened to a LeBron James trainer interview where they talked about solely eating organic—no sports drinks, no fast food, nothing. That dude is a monster on the court, so take note people! I'm thankful for athletes like Tom Brady who share these truths, Kobe Bryant who is a part of Body Armor (a much better Gatorade), and the many others who are speaking the truth and sharing their connection between success and lifestyle choices. This does not only pertain to organic eating, working out, and the right "team;" it is also about mindset. We will talk more about this in *Mindfulness, Meditation, and Mindsets.*

For the most part, our family has been supportive. At the same time, like normal grandparents, ours feel the need to "treat" our kids or give them things I don't give them. It can even get to the point where they think our kids are missing out. There certainly has to be a respectful, ongoing conversation, especially when it comes to allergies, sensitivities, and behaviors.

A lot of things make me cringe on the inside, but for the sake of relationship and peace, I keep a lot of thoughts to myself. Thankfully, my parents, sister, and mother-in-law all eat organic.

They also go out of their way to ensure they respect our food boundaries at family gatherings or when they have my kids over. It took a lot of time and a lot of tears, as learning to navigate those waters can be tricky and tense at times.

So it's not perfect, and it is still a process, especially when it comes to food allergies and not just preferences. All of our kids have some intolerance, sensitivity, or gene mutation. So all this isn't just about personal lifestyle choices; it is about their health. Yes, people have told me *this or that is not going to kill them,* or *it's not going to kill you.* Sure, they might be right, it's not going to kill anyone. But it may give us a headache. It may give us a nasty attitude where we don't feel our best selves. It may give us a stomachache or brain fog. It may give us a rash on our back (yes, that's happened a time or two). It may make us break out on our face. How about those tiny little bumps on the back of your arms? Yep, gluten. It might give us an itchy scalp or breakout. It may give us a cough or cold. Who knows? What we do know is that it affects us.

> *"Before you heal someone, ask him if he's willing to give up the things that made him sick."*
> — *Hippocrates*

One of my sons can suffer terribly from food-sensitivity migraines and emotional outbursts. (Yes, it's a thing!) He is doing better about making choices, but it's tough when he's in environments where pizza and candy are fully accessible—and being a teenage boy, good luck with that! I've also had to do a lot of letting go and letting my kids make their own choices to find out on their own that their decisions have consequences. My kids have had to learn that it's up to them how they want to feel physically, emotionally, and mentally. And how they feel doesn't just pertain to their food choices, but their friend choices, media choices, and heart choices. At times I know I've come off crazy to my husband and family, and I've explained to them that it's not just about my convictions, my allergies, or my calling, but it's me wanting the best for the people I love.

There is always a way to talk to those who we care about and love. Here's the deal, do we want to give them the information and resources at the diagnosis? Of course, we do! And sadly, many times they are not open to any other options until the diagnosis comes. But what if we could get people to be proactive before the diagnosis and make simple choices?

Even just following my Ten Keys to Wholeness in *Next Level Living* would make a huge difference in families, communities, schools, and athletes. When I hear daily from customers about their emergency gallbladder surgery, their tumor, their disability, the number of meds they are on, and the skin issues they are having, I realize how real this is. How many people are suffering? How could they have prevented those things? How many people have been sold and slimed by medical systems? It only makes this fire inside me burn stronger, and it causes me to realize what a gift *health* is daily. It drives me (yes, to be annoying and crazy at times) to want the best for those I love and for the future generation to come. It's going to be a sad world with fewer innovations and creations if most people are sick, medicated, or suffering in some way. It doesn't have to be this way.

It's going to take a lot more than you and me choosing wisely. It's going to take an overhaul of systems, to say the least. It's not impossible though. One day, one choice, one person, one dollar, one word, and one truth at a time. Each of us has a story, a journey, and a path. I honor you right where you are.

IT'S A PROCESS

Now hear me, just because you eat exclusively organic, have a non-toxic home, and do all the things, doesn't mean you're promised perfect health. Why?

1. We have so many environmental toxins.
2. We don't detox correctly or as often as we should.
3. A lot of us have stored-up toxins, dormant viruses, and unknown allergies.
4. We "abused our bodies" for years and decades.
5. We can have scarring and damage that isn't always felt or seen.
6. There are emotional wounds and traumas along with mindsets we have not yet dealt with.
7. We live in a fallen and broken world.

I say this to be honest and to drive home the value of a lifestyle and not stopping once you make changes. I have been personally digging deeper into my own health, even though I feel amazing. I have dealt with some hormone things (years ago I had fibroids), I have done gallbladder flushes, ran blood work, and tested for things I didn't even know were a thing, like lectins and lipids. I still want to know more about my genome. I'm still discovering, and as I head toward my forties, I want to be healthier and stronger than ever (for the record, I feel better in my thirties than in my twenties). I want to know my markers and my body. I would encourage you to do the same, no matter what part of the journey you are on.

At the beginning of 2019, I sent my blood work to Dr. Hilu, one of the world's top cellular health doctors. He has machines and systems that don't even compare to what's available in America. This is a *cellular* blood test! It's next level, and I highly suggest it.

He found thirteen imbalances of a possible eight hundred and eighty-four (yes, that's how deep this test is). All my standard panels from the previous two years showed normal ranges and none of these imbalances. He said my system is clean and my body loves the "diet" I'm on. Of the thirteen imbalances, I'm already treating and taking supports for six of them, and the others I started treating right away. I really thought there was nothing for me to change or do! I was wrong, and I'm grateful for it.

About half of the imbalances are connected to my gene mutation and celiac disease, but one of the findings was shocking to me. It is connected to the silent enemy of environmental toxins, my childhood (vaccines, food, and silver filings), and my mother's womb. Did you know that heavy metals and the result of a poor diet are passed down to you in the womb, and your womb environment still affects you today? A recent epigenetic study showed that they found memories in DNA from fourteen generations back. Crazy, right?

Dr. Hilu also suggested I avoid all types of stress and relational conflict to help with some of these imbalances. As a mom of three and a business owner, we know that isn't exactly possible. What I will do instead is go for more massages, take more full self-care days, increase my meditation and self-compassion, and take a few more soul-nourishing trips.

Even though you feel amazing and have great sleep, energy, skin, digestion, immune system, and clear focus doesn't mean something isn't going on. My cellular blood work is proof of that. These types of tests are a major key to prevention. It might not be that something is a full-blown issue just yet, but finding out about a potential issue can help you prevent it with a holistic treatment plan. If you can't work with someone like this, I strongly encourage individualized care within the functional medicine realm so you can get real answers and an effective plan in place. Even if you're like me and you already do *all the things,* it still matters, and it is important.

Everyone is different and what works for Virginia or for me might not be for you. I give you permission to discover, explore, and try to find the best things for you. This road is not meant to be walked alone. Get the support, help, answers, and truth you need. You don't know how good you can feel until you *feel good.*

Do you know what is even more powerful than our choices and voices? *Our bodies!* God knew what He was doing when He created these amazing, complex, creative systems that all have a purpose. Your body can heal, and your mind can heal; they were *made* to heal! Yes, many of us have consumed years worth of chemicals, toxins (mental and emotional), and slowly, unknowingly poisoned ourselves and our homes. As a result, all those factors have affected us in different ways. Each one of us is unique, and as much as there are general foundations to health, we need individualized care and strategies. *Everyone* can benefit from following some core foundations and upgraded choices, of course.

This is not an overnight fix; this is a lifelong journey and process we get to surrender to and be a part of. It takes your body a full six months to completely eliminate gluten and grains from your system. Sugar and conventional dairy take three weeks to ninety days. The compound buildup in our livers, gallbladders, digestive systems, neural pathways, nervous systems, hearts, minds, blood, and beyond will take time, friends. This is not to overwhelm or discourage you, but to let you know there is a process, and there will be days it's hard.

Having a strong "why" is going to be essential to keeping disciplined during the detox, purge, and shift. At times, it will seem easier to go through that drive-thru or buy the same familiar things. Don't. We are powerful to choose. We are powerful to take knowledge and put it into action. We are powerful to share this journey with others. Never underestimate the power of your journey, your story, and your voice. Please know many are walking this road with you; you are not alone.

CHAPTER TWO

A DAY IN MY HOLISTIC LIFE

MY GENERAL DAILY ROUTINE

"Legendary leaders have legendary mornings."

Routines and rituals are oxygen to productivity. I would not be able to run a successful family, business, podcast, write a book, speak, be this healthy and happy, and live my best life without them. Routine is your friend. I'm not saying you don't leave room for a mental health day, a spontaneous get-away, or intentional leisure. I have found the more automated my life is, the more time I've spent aligning myself in the first hour of the morning. The more I have delegated and elimi-nated the right things, my energy, creativity, time, and health have increased. Assuming things will just happen or change organically is a passive excuse not to start implementing. Be allergic to average! Please commit to a legendary and epic routine so you can have an epic and legendary life.

> **"To have the rewards that very few have,**
> **do the things that very few people are willing to do."**
> — *Robin Sharma*

I have always (depending on the season of life) followed a principle of "tithing" my morning. I take the first hour to get up before the kids to align my mind, body, and spirit. As of January 2019, I elevated that by joining the 5 AM Club. Robin Sharma and his book, *The 5 AM Club*, came into my life and helped confirm the importance of this and even gave it a formula.

First sixty minutes of your day:
20 minutes *sweat*
20 minutes *reflect and meditate*
20 minutes *learn*
Undistracted. While the world sleeps, you strengthen your life. To be great, one must practice great disciplines. The key here is no electronics. As Robin Sharma says, "Own your morning. Elevate your life."

I tweak the principle slightly and practice:
15-20 minutes *journal, prayer, intentions, visualization, and daily devotion*
45-60 minutes (at gym) *listen to podcast or TED Talk while working out. Close with meditation in the sauna.*
15-20 minutes *post gym nutrient-dense meal or Bulletproof coffee, read, and meditate (without an app)*

4:50 AM Alarm goes off (a song, not a preset sound).

4:55 AM Set binaural tones to morning setting. Journal and write dreams, "Thankfuls," and "I Am" declarations. Make the bed. Set intentions for the day. Talk with God and "check in" (self-compassion).

5:15 AM Personal care routine: clean tongue, brush teeth, use face roller, and put on tallow. Drink 8-20oz of lemon and chlorophyll water. (I use a Hydro Flask and make sure my water is room temperature.)

5:20 AM Head to gym. Take phone off airplane mode. Turn on binaural tones and podcast.

5:30 AM Gym. Depending on the day, I will do anything from cardio, weights, spin, TRX, or yoga. I listen to an audiobook, podcast, or TED Talk while working out. One to two times a week I do something active outdoors instead of at the gym.

6:20 AM Sauna and meditation using Soultime or Headspace app.

6:40 AM Start breakfast and wake up kids. Eat breakfast and take supplements. Apply and diffuse essential oils. Get everyone aligned and off for the day.

7:15 AM Leave house. School carpool. Speak life over my kids and ask them what they are thankful for. Prayer time for our day together.

7:55 AM Arrive back home.

8:00 AM Tidy up. Read Bible (I love my paper copy of The Passion Translation), journal, and meditate while enjoying coffee.

8:30 AM Prep dinner. Check messages and personal email. Check in with hubby.

8:45 AM Check business and kids' school messages on GroupMe, Marco Polo, and social media. Post on social media (I mostly post using the preset Planoly). Check emails on laptop. (I don't have my work email on my phone.)

Drink more water (all day).

9:15 AM Depending on the day, I'm either at Eco Chic or doing focused and productive work at home, such as creating, book-keeping, orders, vendors, and invoices. The first ninety minutes are deeply focused, undistracted, and poured into important work. (One morning a week, I meet friends to hike, walk, and pray from 8:00 AM to 9:00 AM. One morning a month, I have a women's small group brunch.)

> **12:00 PM** Take a break to stand, play with Zoe (our English Lab who is on a completely raw paleo diet from SmallBatch), go outside, eat, and check in on social media. This is also when I do my mid-day meditation, get some sun, and be outside for about fifteen minutes.

> **1:00 PM** Creative work on days I work at home (marketing, writing, recording).

3:00 PM Pick up kids from school. Carpool, sports, snacks, and more dinner prep. Tidy up and family check in. Listen to another podcast.

I'll usually have a kombucha or herbal drink between 3:00 PM and 5:00 PM.

5:00 - 6:30 PM Family dinner and family chores. Check in on social media, emails, and tasks depending on sports schedules. Family time.

7:00 PM Next day prep (lunches, outfits, homework, and check-list). Connect with each person who is home. Run through my week or next day.

8:00 PM Wind down. No phone (this can be hard at times), turn on binaural tones, apply Serenity essential oil, and diffuse oils. Take CBD (if it was a high-stress day) and magnesium. Use face oil and jade roller on face and neck. Meditate and reflect. Text myself my to-do lists and priorities for the next day. Read. Turn phone on airplane mode (unless my kids aren't home or I'm on-call for a birth).

9:00 - 10:00 PM Sleep supports. (See *Holistic Must-Haves and Pantry Swaps.*) Go to sleep. My ideal sleep time and circadian rhythm is 9:30 PM to 4:45 AM, and I get that sweet spot at least once a week.

On weekends I still practice the 5 AM Club one of the days. The other day, I still practice my 20/50/20 over extended coffee and reading, and it usually begins at 6:00 AM or 7:00 AM. Most Sundays (as long as I'm not away at sports or working) are spent prepping and planning meals, backpacks, outfits, and doing laundry. We also recharge with family time and rest time (journaling, reading, being outdoors, and writing), and attend church.

MY HOLISTIC HABITS

Food and Wellness:
I drink green juice or celery juice. (Celery juice in the morning is a great practice.)
I drink bone broth.
I drink dandelion tea two times a week.
I drink fire cider and chaga five days a week.
I take wellness shots.
We use a Berkey filter for our water.
I use superfoods and mushrooms (i.e., Organifi, Ancient Nutrition, Moodbeli, Four Sigmatic).

We use cast iron for cooking.

I am not Danielle Walker, but I read her books, and they are my favorite go-to cookbooks.

Everything I eat is organic. Yes, 99.9 percent of *everything.*

I eat clean; I subscribe to a primal paleo diet.

I do not eat gluten, grains, refined sugar, legumes, or dairy unless it's raw, grass-fed dairy.

I get most of my staple food items from Thrive Market.

I take daily supplements. (See page 47 for a list of what works for my body, hormones, age, and blood type. There are many factors that go into what specific supplements I take. A general rule for any age is to start by taking vitamin D3, a probiotic, and magnesium.)

As a creature of ritual and routine, I will confess, I repeat a lot of the same meals and foods, but it works for me. Considering there are a million meal plans, shopping lists, and snack idea boards on Pinterest, I won't be sharing too much here. There are amazing authors and health coaches you can connect with that live for all things food, meal prep, and Instant Pots.

Typical Daily Meals and Snacks:

I fast 7:00 PM to 7:00 AM almost daily. If I have something later, it's a spoon of raw honey, almond butter, or a banana.

Breakfast: Organic, local, pasture-raised eggs with hot sauce. Once a week, as a treat, I'll have hemp bread or a Canyon Bakehouse bagel. I drink a Bulletproof or adaptogen coffee. I also have a piece of fruit. I rotate buckwheat cereal, protein pancakes, paleo waffles, sweet potato breakfast bowls, kefir with honey, and fruit throughout the week, as well. Breakfast is my biggest meal of the day.

Snack: Nuts, fruit, dried fruit, grass-fed meat stick, hard-boiled egg, nut butter packet, cut up vegetables, or a paleo bar. I also eat a few squares of dark chocolate every day per my midwife's orders. They're paleo (dairy-free, gluten-free, soy-free, grain-free, refined sugar-free), and it's packed with clean energy and magnesium. Winning at life over here.

<u>Lunch:</u> Usually leftovers, salad, or something way easy (like an avocado with raw cheese or Applegate organic lunch meat and apples with almond butter). Sometimes I'll just have a quick bar.

<u>Dinner:</u> I don't eat a big dinner, but it's usually some type of vegetable and a small amount of meat, and maybe a carb, like a sweet potato. I often have some type of eggs, breakfast food, or broth for dinner, depending on what I made for my family. I cook three or four nights per week, and we meal plan.

What I Eat When Eating Out:
I don't eat out a lot.
I eat at allergy-friendly places.
I communicate that I have an allergy, not a preference.
I ask if they can use olive oil, coconut oil, or offer raw veggies.
I always have food in my bag, or I eat before.
I have packets of my own mustards, crackers, and sweeteners.
I bring organic digestive enzymes, Digestzen roller, and activated charcoal.

Meat and Produce I Purchase:
Be Love Farm
Butcher Box
Casa Rosa Farm
Eatwell Farm
Lockewood Acres
Nugget Markets
Sprouts Farmers Market
Thrive Market
Whole Foods

Supplements I Take Daily:
Adrenal support (ashwagandha and holy basil)
B-complex

Brain Octane Oil (in my coffee)
Camu camu
Chlorella
Collagen (in my coffee)
Colloidal silver (at least once a week)
Curcumin (post blood work results)
Fermented cod liver oil (omegas)
Glutamine (post blood work results)
Glycine (post blood work results)
Immune supports (more info listed on the following pages and in *Holistic Must-Haves and Pantry Swaps.* I especially take these if I'm feeling under the weather or during wintertime.)
Maca root with selenium
Magnesium
Manuka honey 13+ (at least once a week)
Methyl B12
Methyl folate
Multi-mushroom blend
Nootropics (brain and focus support)
Probiotics
Raw vitamin C
Revive Multi
Silica
Spirulina
Superfood blend
Vitamin D3

Energy and Focus Supports:
Brain Octane Oil
Coffee (it has polyphenols and increases BDNF)
Essential oils (peppermint)
Exercise (Here's a thought: *What if every time you were stressed, instead of snacking you exercised?*)
Lots of water with lemon

Mindset, heart, and spirit health
Methyl B12
Nootropics
Superfood blend
Vitamin B-complex

Stress Supports:
Adaptogens
CBD (THC-free)
Essential oils
Magnesium
Multi-mushroom blend

Sleep Supports:
CBD (THC-free)
Essential oils
Sleep practices (see in *Fat, Addicted, Tired, Stressed, Broke, and Sick*)

Immune Supports:
Bone broth
Colloidal silver
Echinacea
Elderberry
Extra probiotics
Fire cider
Goldenseal
High dose of vitamin C
Kefir
Manuka honey 13+
On Guard essential oil
Oregano essential oil
Propolis
Zinc

<u>Supplements My Kids Take:</u>
Camu camu or vitamin C
Collagen (only my oldest son)
Omegas (fermented cod liver oil)
Probiotics
Vitamin D3
Magnesium

<u>Personal Care:</u>
I have and use an Ōura ring.
I wear blue light blocking glasses.
I use red light therapy.
I use a jade roller every night and put a drop of Serenity essential oil on my temples and neck before bed.
I diffuse Citrus Bliss, Serenity, frankincense, lavender, or vetiver essential oils.
I take essential oils and herbs.
I get my blood work done at least every few years. (I suggest using your holistic practitioner, Andrea Thompson, or Dr. Hilu.)
I go to the chiropractor twice a month, and sometimes weekly. (I have zero back issues.)
I get regular massages and facials (using only organic products).
I work out four to six days a week and go in the sauna at least three days a week.
I stretch or do slow flow yoga weekly.
I play volleyball. (I like to think I'm on the USA team, but it's really just city ball.)
I make sure to get at least ten to twenty minutes of sun each day when possible.
I do a foot detox at a wellness center once a year. Home foot detoxes work great, too.
I do detox baths, but not as often as I would like as I don't have a tub.

Beauty and Skincare Products I Use:
Eco Tan
GingerChi (jade roller)
Gold Clover
Innersense Beauty
Luminance
Mud Mouth
PAAVANI Ayurveda
Prana Brush
Skinny & Co.
Thinksport
100% Pure

"Victims love entertainment, leaders love knowledge."
— *Robin Sharma*

Self-Development:
Educate. Educate. Educate.
I am always learning.
I attend a conference of some kind at least once every three months.
I listen to at least ten podcasts every week.
I read ten to fourteen books each year.
I watch documentaries.
I hire coaches.

Mental Health:
I have mentors.
I have a tribe and I'm in community.
I do sound therapy.
I practice gratitude, intentions, and meditation.
I use the 20/20/20 principle with social media.
> I take twenty minutes in the morning, twenty in the afternoon, and twenty in the evening to go on social media strategically. I answer DMs, comments, post, and enjoy content

from encouraging leaders on health and spirituality. I don't follow pop culture accounts or anything negative. I unfollow and mute 75 percent of people on my social media. I also make sure a few close friends are not muted so I can also engage with them. You could also do that in two thirty-minute sessions, or one full hour a day. The goal is not to use social media for more than one hour each day.

I apply time management, time blocking, and goal setting to my daily life.

I go on a monthly field trip out of town to explore, shop local, get inspired, and enjoy organic food made at small businesses.

I practice disconnected days.

I practice breathwork and earthing (grounding).

I hike and travel.

I practice self-compassion.

At Home:

Our entire home is organic and non-toxic.

Our lightbulbs are non-LED.

We don't have a smart meter.

We have our WiFi box set to turn off from midnight to 5:00 AM every day.

We have a garden. It's definitely a work in progress—we did enjoy the forty-two berries we got last summer. (Call me Joanna Gaines.)

I burn sage or herbal bundles. (It's proven to get bacteria out of the air.)

We use salt lamps and SafeSleeves for EMF reduction.

We use bath ball filters to get toxins out of bath water. A better option would be a whole house reverse osmosis system.

We don't use fabric softeners or dryer sheets.

We use organic pest care; *never* Roundup.

A lot of our furniture is Restoration Hardware or WHdesign. We strive for sustainable and non-toxic.

If we paint, we use low VOC or non-toxic paint.

I'd love to say we compost, but we are not there yet. We only have one bag of trash per week for a family of five, and we fill our recycle bin.

We reuse as much as possible, and mason jars are the cup of choice.

We don't use a microwave. A stove, toaster oven, and convection oven work great.

We buy local, small, give-back, and fair trade as much as possible.

I buy homemade and handmade before I ever make it myself.

In eight years of owning a store, we haven't bought paper once.

All cleaning products and hygiene products are organic and mostly homemade.

For the record, I have three total cleaners in my house:

1. Bac-Out—all things stain and cleaning
2. Vinegar and water with essential oils
3. Rockin Green laundry soap and sports spray. *It works!*

I also use Norwex cloths for windows and stainless-steel surfaces.

I buy second-hand often. When it's new, my rules are:

1. It must be meaningful, minimal, and sustainable.
2. I have to get rid of two items to get the new one.

I need to mention that not all vitamins are real or effective. You want to look for organic, cellular, food- and herb-based, as well as a reputable company, like B Corps. The best vitamins will come from functional medicine facilities, certified health stores, and certified health coaches. According to the Organic Consumers Association, some of the synthetic materials in synthetic vitamins come from coal tar derivatives, the same toxins that cause throat cancer in tobacco smokers. Commercial vitamins are a scam and waste of money; they will go right through you and most have additives, coloring, fillers, and other things (soy, gluten, sugar). If you see chloride, hydrochloride, acetate, or nitrate on the list of ingredients, the manufacturer used synthetics for the product. Just as you check the ingredient list in foods you buy, you should always check the ingredients in your vitamins.

Another red flag when purchasing vitamins is that you don't want them to be exposed to harsh temperatures (too hot or too cold), as this can destroy the cells. Many vitamins might sit in trucks or warehouses (i.e., Amazon), and you might think you got a good deal, but the supplement company won't warranty it due to temperature concerns and knock-offs. Yes, Amazon sells fake vitamins and oils. Buying directly from the company or from a trusted retailer is your best bet. Ideally, your vitamins will come in dark, glass containers or toxin-free bioplastic. You should also consider where you store your vitamins to ensure they don't get damaged.

Now that you know my entire day, I'd like to speak to yours. As much as this works for me, you might find something works better for you. I suggest you at least try something similar, and maybe curated to your life, for a minimum of sixty-six days before you give up on it. When you own your morning, own your decisions, own your thoughts, and own your actions, you can own your life.

CHAPTER THREE

THE POWER OF PEACE, LOVE, AND GRATITUDE

THE PART YOU DIDN'T KNOW YOU NEEDED

"You can eat the kale, hit the gym, drink the water, and take the vitamins, but if you don't deal with the S&^% going on in your heart and head, you're still going to be unhealthy."

Guys, as much as I love eating healthy, taking the right supplements for my body, being in community, living my passion and purpose, working out, and enjoying life, I still get to deal with my heart. Hello. I'm human. I have teenagers. I'm a woman. I'm a wife. I'm a daughter, friend, sister, and leader. There is pain. There is disappointment. There is failure. There is betrayal. There is pressure. There is stress. There are hurtful words. No doubt.

I know you want examples, so here are a few without names and details because, for the love, it's not a biography, amen? You have a brilliant imagination of what this would look like, and then some.

I have had employees accuse me of crazy things because they were let go due to unethical behaviors. Employees have stolen from me and tried everything to see me and my business fail. I have had what I thought were ride-or-die best friends turn on me for their gain, a new opportunity, used me for my knowledge, generosity, resources, and kindness. I have had "trolls" write death threats, publicly post lies about me or my family all over social media and Yelp because of my religious, political, and health views. I've had people I deeply love and care for, who were in the trenches with me, move thousands of miles away, where I then laid bricks alone until God brought new partnerships.

My parents had me at sixteen. I had my whole twelve-year-old safe world shattered when my parents made decisions in direct conflict to the way I was raised. I rebelled from my faith from ages thirteen to sixteen and made choices that caused me and others deep pain. My children have made decisions or aligned themselves with people I would never choose.

I have been left at the worst of times. I've been broke, in debt, shared a car, and used WIC to buy groceries. I've had dark seasons in my marriage of almost eighteen years. I married at the age of nineteen and became a mother at the age of twenty. That alone is a book for another day. I've been judged for being influential, outspoken, and taking a risk. I've had people reject me and my ideas because they were intimidated by my confidence. I've been told, "*No, that's a bad idea,*" to then see it done but under another name. I have been laughed at for my courage and my faith. I have been mocked. I have been verbally abused. I have been emotionally neglected. I lost my uncle who was a second dad to me, a mentor, and an inspiration, taken far too young.

I've lost business deals, contracts, and money. I've had a dear friend throw years of mentorship and friendship away while believing someone who used, lied, broke contracts, and set out to sabotage my business in the name of fame and personal gain. I've had threats and verbal attacks as a government official in hopes of me resigning my position because people are afraid of the truth and change. I've had my ideas copied (but they can't steal your spirit though... *Okayyyy!*). I've had many eleventh hours and God-if-you-don't-come-through moments in my life. I know pain. I know rejection. I know abandonment. I know neglect. I know disappointment. I know criticism. I know fear.

I also know healing, hope, health, freedom, confidence, forgiveness, truth, and power. I realize many of you have been through far more and much worse. I acknowledge I have had an overall great life, for sure. My parents are amazing and huge supporters. They are my friends, and they restored their hearts, marriage, lives, and faith through years of deep work.

I think this is where we miss it in our culture. If it's not "this big" or "this traumatic," we minimize it. That only causes more pain and shame. Why can't we validate, empathize, and extend compassion instead of comparing and criticizing the level of someone's grief? It doesn't matter how much, how long, or how bad. What matters is what someone feels. Can we do better? Can we seek to understand and validate? I'm not saying allow anyone to be a victim and let them stay in their pit—not one bit. I am saying let's listen, let's love, let's hold space, and let's check in.

> **"Gratitude is not only the greatest of virtues,**
> **but the parent of all others."**
> **— *Cicero***

For me, using tools like the daily 20/50/20 method, self-compassion, journaling, reading the Bible (The Passion Translation is my favorite), being in community and held accountable, staying active, meditation, prayer, worship, and having a legit high standard in my atmospheres (my home, my car, my business) with media and all mediums. I'm doing the work. I can usually rise above, forgive quickly, or interpret other people's stuff (projection and gaslighting), but not always. Because #life.

Cultivating and protecting peace is everything. Making margin to deal with the stuff is important, too. Guys, protecting your peace does not have to be candles, yoga mats, and sage sticks. (Though I love me some of that.) It can be three minutes in the car in the driveway. It can be with a good side of CBD and your favorite stress aromatherapy roller. It can be a ten-minute walk. A five-minute letter to "Dear *(hurt part of you)*." A text or phone call to a trusted friend or mentor. Another way to protect our peace, keep our love on, and stay thankful is to guard what we are listening to, watching, following, and consuming on social media.

PEACE, LOVE, GRATITUDE

"Health is not just about what you're eating.
It's also about what you're thinking and saying."

When I speak on love, I don't just mean for life, God, and others. I mean self-love, too, which we will talk about more later. Sometimes I can do all of that (within my control), and then I have an unhinged customer come in, or a teenager project onto me and let me know how much I am failing at motherhood, and on and on the list goes.

And then what? Yes, resort back to the tools I mentioned, so when you're practicing them daily, the hits don't feel as bad (which is fantastic), but you're also aware that you get to choose. You get to choose to believe what someone is saying or not. One of my favorite practices is *RRRR: reject, rebuke, replace, release.* I do this with every lie or negative thought, as well as when things get thrown at me or my business.

The very first and most powerful thing to remember is that *it is a choice.* You are powerful to choose. You actually have control over your thoughts, feelings, words, food, and financial choices. *You are powerful.*

We have conditioned ourselves to lean one way or the other. It is possible to condition yourself to believe the best, be strong, have peace, extend love, and be deeply grateful no matter what you're facing. I promise you I showed up, recorded a podcast, written a blog post, spoken on stage, prayed for someone, or served at Eco Chic while I was in the middle of a lot of toxic conversations and words. Yes, there were moments I cried in my car before hitting the store or the stage, moments I took a deep breath and spoke an affirmation (that I believed) and carried on until I could do deeper work.

Have you ever known someone who had nothing, faced the fire of hell, and then they had everything and many blessings, yet they were the same person? It's possible. People can also remain victims, though; people can choose pain. People can run circles around lies, hurts, wounds, pain, and failure instead of taking every problem and making it a purpose, and every mess a message. It's a choice.

What I'm not saying is *Don't feel. Feelings aren't real. Shove it and get over it.* I don't believe in piling, shoving, repressing, ignoring, or lying. There is a real process of dealing with hurts, emotions, and disappointments. Cry. Feel. Be mad. Be sad. Just don't stay there. Peace and happiness are inside jobs. (Thanks Bill Johnson and Kris Vallotton for teaching this for decades.) And *joy* isn't the same thing as happiness. Let that simmer for a minute. Let it cool, then digest it.

HEALING HURTS

"The more you express gratitude for what you have, the more likely you will have even more to express gratitude for."
— *Zig Ziglar*

What happens when we decide not to feel, heal, and forgive? We turn to anger, addiction, avoidance, abuse/abusing, or avoidance. So how do you heal hurts? (I *firmly* believe in therapy and daily maintenance. This chapter is not a magic wand.)

1. Use the *RRRR* method.
2. Have self-compassion (see list in *The Power of Self*).
3. Forgive.
4. Cry. *Yep, it's good to cry.*
5. Guard your thoughts, mind, and words. Know what you're feeding yourself.
6. Pray and meditate.
7. Find an affirmation, verse, or quote you can put on your mirror, in your car, or as your phone background.
8. Share with a mature, trusted mentor or friend.
9. Seek counseling or therapy.
10. Ask yourself about repetitive pains or triggers. *When did this start? When did I first feel it?* Go back to that place for deeper healing. Take note if you're staying in a wound or trigger for more than three minutes. If you are, then, as my mentor taught me, you need to look deeper.
11. Don't shove, bury, pile, repress, or ignore, physically and spiritually. *This is how we store toxic emotions, and they block us from breakthrough and blessing.* Please process, feel, and express emotions.
12. Self-care (see list in *The Power of Self*).

I realize this is much deeper than a few pages in a book and I want to give place to your very real pain, trauma, disappointment, fears, and tears. They matter. What you have seen, been through, and dealt with matters. I want to say I am sorry for the pain you have experienced: the rejections, betrayals, lies, abandonment, fears, and lonely days. It's no wonder things have been hard—look at all you have endured. It's no wonder people don't understand—you have been through so much. I validate your pain, your purpose, your feelings, your hurts, your traumas, and your disappointment. You are seen. You matter. You are not alone. Your pain and hurts are valid. I am so sorry for the residual effects of this deep hurt.

As a woman of faith, I am always going to circle back to Jesus. For me, this is the beginning, the end, the everything. You don't have to understand or agree, but this is my belief. As much as I love, use, and support all—and I mean *all*—the tools, I also know God can heal in a moment what takes years. He is the God of more than enough, the God of hope, the God of healing, the God who restores, the God who hears, the God who saves, the God who answers, the God who protects, the God who provides, the God who makes all things new, the God that moves mountains, and for my fellow Elevation fans, *yes*, we will see Him do it again. I'll be sharing more about this theology in *Dear Christians*.

Wholeness is where this book is a bit different. We are not putting all our chips on faith alone, or exercise alone, or prayer alone, or organic food alone, or mindsets alone. This is a lifestyle that engages every part. Mind. Body. Spirit. Emotions. They *all* matter.

> *"Abundance will flow into our life when gratitude flows out of our heart."*
> — *Jon Gordon*

The Power of Gratitude:
adjective
1. warmly or deeply appreciative of kindness or benefits received; thankful: *I am grateful to you for your help.*
2. expressing or actuated by gratitude: *a grateful letter.*
3. pleasing to the mind or senses; agreeable or welcome; refreshing: *a grateful breeze.*

Scientific studies have shown that those who practice gratitude sleep better. Thankfulness is a superpower and a core key to health. It is *impossible* to be miserable and thankful at the same time. I'm not a gratitude expert, but I know what we focus on magnifies. If someone does something to hurt or upset you, it's easy to step into our ego and highlight all the negative—which only feeds your pain and distance—instead of choosing to lean into yourself and see the good, believe the best, accept, and forgive. This is mostly applied within the home with family. Don't we all know it? What if we did more acknowledging versus focusing on the failures? Now, I can totally pick up on your thoughts right about now:

But... that will justify their poor behavior.
But... that will let them get away with it.
But... that will make them think I'm okay with this.
But... that will not teach them anything.
But... they must suffer and pay for the pain they have caused.
But... shall I go on?

Guess what? Worry about you. Yes, it's essential to communicate how we feel, and what we need in a "hero-sandwich" way. I'm a *huge* believer in communicating how we feel. However, it doesn't always mean that people are where we hope they would be. Again, we are now holding toxic emotions, and these things wear down our immune and nervous systems. There have been tons of studies about physical health and the connection to our emotional health. I haven't met a bitter, angry person who beams with light and joy, have you? You can feel and see it on someone's countenance.

Thankful people are present.
Thankful people are happy.
Thankful people are content.
Thankful people make the most of every moment.
Thankful people are purpose-led.

Thankful people are centered.
Thankful people are generous.
Thankful people are healthy.

You will always get back what you give and then some. In quantum physics, everything you say and put out looks for its match or a mirror to come back. (Okay, pause a moment—I'm not an expert or scientist and can hardly spell neural or quantum without spell check.) Gratitude isn't just good manners. However, never underestimate the power of a *thank you*. I'm so *pro*-thank you cards, thank you texts, thank you snacks, thank you coffee, thank you chocolate, thank you high-fives—all of it.

Thankfulness, thankful, and *thanks* are mentioned in the Bible over a hundred times. When you are grateful for the things in your life—big and small—you always seem to find more things to be grateful for.

People, and especially critics, will say, "It's easy for you to be thankful, you have *this* or *that*." I'd like to call BS on that. There are plenty of thankful people with little, less, and worse. I can share many examples, but one of my favorites is my dear friend, Terces. She lived in a yurt and washed dishes with a hose and bucket. She was just as happy and powerful then as she is now, living in a beautifully built farmhouse on that same property.

Thankful people who are in difficult places inspire us. To name a few: Inky Johnson. Nick Vujicic. My son's friend who lost his dad and brother, then within two years, his mom was in a horrific accident. My friend, Andrea, who overcame cancer, trauma, and much more. She uses her life to serve and inspire others. Many people I know and admire have come from pain, adversity, and setbacks, yet they remain thankful and positive.

"Gratitude as an attitude of the heart has nothing to do with what you have or what you don't have."
— Brian Buffini

Anyone can be thankful right now with where they are and what they have. It is very similar to the principle of giving: if you won't give when you have little, what makes you think you will give when you have more? If you're not thankful now, what makes you think you will be thankful later? There is also an assumption that people with "more" are happier and more grateful, but that is not always the fact. I believe those with healthy mindsets, heartsets, and spiritsets will be trusted with *more*. And *more* means something a little different to everyone.

How to Practice and Increase Gratitude:

1. Keep a gratitude journal or notebook. Practice writing at least three things every morning and at least three more at night. (Ten is an excellent goal.)
2. When something hard or negative happens, find the good in it, and turn that energy into prayer, positivity, and gratitude. Even speak out loud *I am thankful for...*
3. Perspective. I have so much to say about this—it's everything.
4. Begin to recount every time you had a breakthrough, answered prayer, miracle, or blessing.
5. Show thankfulness to someone through a card, text, or coffee.
6. Watch how you say things. (I.e., *I have to* versus *I get to. I am* versus *I'll try. I will* versus *maybe.*) Align your mindset with your words, and your words with your mindset.
7. Stay present and be in the moment.

POSITIVITY AND PRODUCTIVITY

"A positive mind is a positive life."

Just saying positive things or putting on a smile isn't enough as your mind, body, and the biofield know the truth. Positivity is an inside job, and it is great friends with true happiness, gratitude, and healthy mindsets. Your mind is a magnet.

Positivity is a key to success, growth, health, peace, and productivity. Positivity affects everything and everyone. Science proves we are wired for love, to believe the best, and to be positive. Dr. Caroline Leaf says this is called the *optimism bias.*

Benefits of Being Positive:

1. Positive people live longer. In a study of nuns, those who regularly expressed positive emotions lived an average of ten years longer than those who didn't.
2. Positive work environments outperform negative work environments.
3. Positive, optimistic salespeople sell more than pessimistic salespeople.
4. Positive leaders are able to make better decisions under pressure.
5. Marriages are much more likely to succeed when the couple experiences a five-to-one ratio of positive to negative interactions, whereas when the ratio approaches a one-to-one ratio, marriages are more likely to end in divorce.
6. Positive people who regularly express positive emotions are more resilient when facing stress, challenges, and adversity.
7. Positive people are able to maintain a broader perspective and see the big picture, which helps them identify solutions, whereas negative people maintain a narrower perspective and tend to focus on problems.
8. Positive thoughts and emotions counter the negative effects of stress. For example, you can't be thankful and stressed at the same time.
9. Positive emotions, such as gratitude and appreciation, help athletes perform at a higher level.
10. Positive people have more friends, which is a key factor in happiness and longevity.
11. Positive and popular leaders are more likely to garner the

support of others and receive pay raises, promotions, and achieve greater success in the workplace.

The Cost of Negativity:

1. According to the Centers for Disease Control and Prevention, 90 percent of doctor visits are stress related.
2. A study found that negative employees can scare off every customer they speak with—for good.
3. At work, too many negative interactions compared to positive interactions can decrease the productivity of a team, according to Barbara Fredrickson's research at the University of Michigan.
4. Negativity affects the morale, performance, and productivity of our teams.
5. One negative person can create a miserable office environment for everyone else.
6. Robert Cross's research at the University of Virginia demonstrates that 90 percent of anxiety at work is created by 5 percent of one's network—the people who zap energy.
7. Negative emotions are associated with decreased life span and longevity.
8. Negative emotions increase the risk of heart attack and stroke.
9. Negativity is associated with greater stress, less energy, and more pain.
10. Negative people have fewer friends.

WHERE DOES POSITIVITY START?

Positivity starts in the thoughts, feelings, and mind. There are a few things we can't control, but the things we can are our thoughts, our feelings, our words, our actions, and our decisions.

Does your mind automatically go to the worst and to being critical of yourself and others (i.e., would have, should have, could have, worry, assumptions, passive thinking, victim mindset)? These thoughts are all run by negativity. When you are a victim, you become your own oppressor. When people don't trust your mood, they don't trust you to lead. Grace always comes before truth. As a leader, we need to have hard conversations, but the way we deliver them should be positive.

Have you ever watched a scary movie and thought, *"Why are they so dumb?"* Studies show that when we are afraid or negative, our brains are dumber. So, to be smarter is to have faith and positivity. If you don't like the word *positivity*, you can use the word *gratitude*, as it's quite impossible to be negative and thankful at the same time. Your attitude about something not only dictates the experience but the effectiveness (aka productiveness). Would you put on depressing, negative music to get some chores done? *No!*

To get really scientific with you, healthy thoughts cause the brain to grow, benefiting your heart health, your muscles, your skin, and your digestive system. Up to 90 percent of illnesses start in the mind with your thoughts.

> *"When we focus on our gratitude, the tide*
> *of disappointment goes out and*
> *the tide of love rushes in."*
> — *Kristin Armstrong*

How to Increase Positivity:
- Believe the best instead of the worst.
- Commit to personal growth and goals.
- Control what you consume (toxic news, toxic foods, negative TV shows, social media).
- Cultivate connection and communication. *Where there is a void, negativity fills space.*
- Do a twenty-one-day brain detox.

- Exercise, journal, meditate.
- Gratitude, gratitude, gratitude.
- Intentional living; be present.
- Love, serve, care.
- Put good stuff in. Take care of yourself.
- Trade every negative narrative for a positive (i.e., identify the lie, limiting belief, or toxic thought, then transmute it).
- Turn complaints into solutions.
- Weed out the negative. *Zero tolerance for complaining; put distance between you and the negative.*

> **"Nothing in the world can bother you as much as your own mind, I tell you. In fact, others seem to be bothering you, but it is not others. It is your own mind."**
> — *Dalai Lama*

Now that you have more of an understanding of the power of peace, love, and gratitude, you can begin to implement these things from the inside out. I will be sharing a lot more around this in-depth a little later.

It's incredible the impact gratitude can have. Whatever you do, resolve today to resist mediocrity and pursue greatness in your mind, body, and spirit. Positivity has the best return on investment. Love always wins. Peace is supreme. A grateful heart is everything.

CHAPTER FOUR

THE SYSTEM IS NOT YOUR FRIEND
(SHOCKING, I KNOW)

"The truth will set you free,
but first it will piss you off."
— *Gloria Steinem*

The system (food, Big Pharma, FDA, and many other organizations) is not your friend. *Say what?* Considering this is a health book, I'm going to skip over the corruption that's invading everything from political (that is very much connected to health), justice, and financial spaces. Don't let nonprofits fool you though. Many of the most well-known are very corrupt at the core. It's real, and we need to be aware, intentional, and awake. As we dig deeper in the next chapter, *Enemies of Health*, you will find there are toxins and chemicals in almost everything.

I share this information with you not to scare you, but to make you aware. This chapter is the part that gets most people, as it should. It's an injustice. It's wrong. Shady. Evil. *Shocking.* And a bit confusing at times. Many times, we find ourselves asking, *"Why are 'they' doing this? What is their goal in all of these toxins and corrupt ways?"* I don't have an exact answer, but I will throw out a few: *power, greed, evil agendas, lack of awareness or knowledge, population control, and broken humanity.*

I must warn you; this section is not made to be taken lightly or skimmed over. Please make sure you create margin to be able to read, process, and reflect on this section. You may need to take extra time for this chapter and take it in bite-sized pieces.

> **"The person hungriest to learn
> will have the most results."**

THE FOOD SYSTEM

I was talking to my husband for a long time about the corruption in our food system before he finally watched *Food Inc.* It was a breakthrough moment for him, as it was for many. We often don't want to know or see the truth, if we are honest. Acknowledging we have been duped or been wrong is hard. The next hard part is actually taking the steps to change and do better. Sometimes people are motivated by a principle or a cause, even more so than for themselves. Whatever gets you there is all that matters. It's not just our food system, but the entire cosmetics, cleaning, education, and healthcare industries. And to be clear, that is not where it stops. I list every ingredient, chemical, and food "issue" in detail in the next chapter, so keep reading to find out the ingredients you want to avoid at all costs.

> **"People are fed by the food industry, which pays
> no attention to our health, and are treated
> by the health industry, which pays
> no attention to food."**
> — *Wendell Berry*

Food companies are cutting corners to increase their bottom line. The ties between Congress and conventional food companies are nothing less than corrupt. Officials from the FDA, EPA, and USDA are often offered high-powered and high-paying jobs with companies that they were assigned to oversee as a government official. We also know "safe reports" have come from "special labs" to get "FDA" approval. Does anyone else see an issue with this? The other issue is the straightforward fact that companies can and do lie. The front of their labels say keywords like "natural" or "real fruit," yet the ingredients show the dye, Red 40, along with corn, soy, sugar, and many other "substances."

When you decide to get fast food, please don't forget that you're really getting dangerous ingredients linked to various cancers and obesity, on top of the fact that it's addicting, unhealthy, and not even real food. In the UK, McDonald's fries have only three ingredients, where in America, there are seventeen. These dangerous ingredients I'm warning you about include MSG, trans fat, sodium nitrite, BHA, BHT, propyl gallate, aspartame, acesulfame-K, olestra, potassium bromate, and food coloring Blue 1 and 2, Red 3, Green 3, and Yellow 6. *Delish.*

Don't even get me started on the treatment of animals and how certain farms are run. I know the vegetarians and vegans reading this get it. Believe it or not, there are happy cows and happy chickens, but they only come from ethically- and organically-run farms. You don't have to be vegetarian or vegan to revolt against these inhumane and unhealthy practices.

If you eat meat, it's crucial you understand organic grass-fed is not the same as organic grass-fed and -finished. When it's just grass-fed, it means they grain-finish the cows instead of letting them be in a pasture (how God intended) to get essential nutrients and sun. If you're avoiding grains, then this is especially an issue. When you are shopping for meat products, you want to look for organic, pasture-raised, local (meat with multiple countries listed is a red flag), and grass-finished.

Another ingredient in meat you want to avoid is *nitrates*. Nitrates are carcinogen preservatives. They are also known to damage cells, and cellular health is everything. Be careful of what the branding looks like, and read the ingredients.

The question is: *Are Americans aware it's not healthy?* I think yes, but I don't think they realize what is really in this unhealthy "food." The other question is: *If we know all of this, why do we keep eating it?* It's likely one of a few things:

1. Self-sabotage. We don't believe we are worthy of taking great care of ourselves or that it even really matters.
2. We are unaware, uninformed, uneducated, and unconscious.
3. Convenience and finances. Note: it's just as easy to toss a bar and an apple into your bag or car daily. It's also cheaper.
4. Addiction. Keep reading to find out why. Studies show food additives are addictive, and we *know* sugar is addictive (it's in everything).
5. Excuses, such as *Well I'm fine,* or *I don't have time,* or *It's not that big of a deal.*

> **"Drugs block our biochemistry to reduce symptoms. Vegetables restore our biochemistry to create health."**
> — *Dr. Terry Wahls*

The goal for these food companies is to make us—their customer and their consumer—dependent on their "drugs" (which some foods *are* drugs: refined sugar). The experts say sugar can be even more addicting than cocaine. Eating sweets block the part in our brain that thinks reasonably and triggers the part that leads to compulsive behavior. We hardwire our brain to crave sugar and eventually build up a tolerance to it! The documentary, *Fed Up*, is another great resource if you want to research this more.

Guys, this is a real thing! By all means, please give your kid some Red Vines and let me know how they act over twenty-four hours. (Shout-out to my 1989 drug dealer, the ice cream man, who always had my goods!) The drugs of choice for me were Red Ropes and Laffy Taffy. And yes, I had a silver crown when I was eight. Thanks, Mom.

As Jason Vale says in *Hungry For Change*, "It's illegal to give a child cigarettes and alcohol, and so it should be, but it's not illegal to give them white, refined sugar or refined fats." This "system" has a plan to get you dumbed down, so you are not woke about what's happening in our world's systems (education, politics, family, media, arts, business, church), and you end up following the herd sick, stressed, quiet, and exhausted. Not to mention you're living in fear and stress because you're not feeling your best and your "diet" consist of the news, heavy metal water, Coffee-Mate, Crisco (I just gagged), Snickers, McDonald's with a side of eczema cream, blood pressure meds, Adderall, and Xanax. On top of all that, all the wounds in our hearts have yet to heal. Many of us are stuck back in our thirteen-year-old rejection, our ten-year-old abandonment, and our sixteen-year-old insecurity. We are great at numbing (yes, that white screen is an issue), shoving, repressing, and projecting, but where does that really get us?

Does this seem like a good plan? Does this feel like your best, rested, healthiest, strongest "you" success plan? I'm thinking no. With this "diet," you are on a path headed to a cheapened life. You need lots of naps, snacks, and pills, to say the least. For the record, I'm not against a good nap and snack. I'm team "Self-Care" all the way. Always. But you must know there is a domino effect in place.

Here is an extreme example: Eat the Standard American Diet (SAD), become addicted, and mindlessly choose food, not fuel. Need drugs and creams. Use chemical products, get cancer, and need chemo. Continue to use chemical products and not understand why you're still not better. Live a low-quality life and experience complications. Repeat. Treat the symptom instead of getting to the root or cause. Silence the symptoms with meds or ignore them and "suddenly" need your gallbladder removed. Never truly heal and get a "free side effect." Get sick and take antibiotics. See your immune system deplete and catch every cold. See increased anxiety and have thyroid or adrenal issues. (Did you know antibiotics stay in your thyroid for seven years and tear your gut apart?) Repeat. Take pills and ruin your liver (to say the least). Watch the news and feel afraid and angry, yet do nothing about it. Repeat. Get offended or hurt so you shove and repress, and wonder why you don't have peace. Repeat. Eat bad food and feel bad. Repeat. I'm pretty sure we get the point now.

A Bloomberg study shows that almost five million Americans get food poisoning every year (that's only the reported ones), and over three thousand people die related to food illness. How and why is this happening in our day and age? How is it that "food" is being approved and sent out like it's "safe" when it's not?

Most Americans are blindly trusting in a system that isn't for them. Think about 2018 and the E. coli outbreaks we experienced. Is it possible this was due to the "sludge" that conventional (non-organic) farms are using? Or is it due to the lack of transparency and coverup of toxins, the liberal use of the word "safe," and the focus being a political gain over personal health? Just a thought.

"Sludge" is what The U.S. Environmental Protection Agency (EPA) calls "biosolids." But what is it really? And why should you care? As an article from *In These Times* explains, sewage sludge is:

> . . . whatever goes into the sewer system and emerges as solids from municipal wastewater treatment plants. Sludge can be (its exact com-

74

position varies and is not knowable) any of the 80,000 synthetic chemicals used by industry; new chemicals created from combining two or more of those 80,000; bacteria and viruses; hospital waste; runoff from roads; pharmaceuticals and over-the-counter drugs; detergents and chemicals that are put down drains in residences; and, of course, urine and feces flushed down toilets.

This toxic stew is sold to farmers who use it to fertilize food crops—a fact most consumers don't know because food producers and retailers aren't required to tell you.

Now what is all the hype about organic, and when did we move away from real food to lab-made crap? It would be a whole lot easier if everything in the store that isn't organic just said *toxic* or *full of chemicals and GMOs* instead of organic needing the labels. Which, by the way, costs organic companies ridiculous amounts of money—so much that it keeps many from going mainstream. Corrupt much? Did you know our current agricultural system has tax dollars paying for the subsidized planting of GMOs, but organic farms have to pay certification fees?

How about non-GMO foods and The Non-GMO Project? Is eating GMO-free enough? How about we start with food additives, as over ten thousand additives are allowed in food. What the kale? Aluminum, artificial colors, BHA and BHT, diacetyl, flavor, propylparaben, potassium bromate, nitrates, and nitrites. Is it just me or does this sound like paint thinner mixed with antifreeze? *Yum.*

Monsanto and Bayer (leading companies in agrochemicals and pharmaceuticals) are facing eight thousand lawsuits because of this. It's an undeniable fact that glyphosate isn't the innocuous agriculture chemical that Monsanto has long claimed. The chemical is known, based on animal, human cell, human epidemiological, and clinical case studies, to damage the liver and kidneys, disrupt hormones, impair reproductive ability, damage gut bacteria, corrupt DNA, and promote cancer. If you're eating GMOs, you're eating Roundup. This is the moment you say, "Oh, that's why she's organic."

How GMOs are Made:

Scientists at Monsanto discovered a strain of bacteria that is herbicide-resistant (Roundup), so they mixed the DNA of that bacteria with food crops. Despite the fact the food is covered in toxic chemicals, the advantage of Roundup is farmers can spray the entire field with herbicide, all the weeds will die, and their food crops will survive. Mixing DNA between two different species is not something that would occur naturally. Most conventional crops come covered in fungicides and pesticides (two carcinogens), compared to a GMO crop that comes wrapped in fungicides, pesticides, and herbicides (three carcinogens)! Which is worse? Two carcinogens or three carcinogens?

If you switch your diet to solely organic for just a week, you will reduce the number of pesticides in your body by *90 percent*. Can I give you a pro-tip? If a label says "natural," it's BS. It is a step in the right direction for a product to be non-GMO *verified*. However, without filling the pages explaining why organic is better, I need to clarify something about GMOs. The issue with non-GMO foods is that they can still be covered in chemicals. Yes, seriously. So when you're shopping for products, look for *organic*. Not natural or non-GMO. If it's organic, it's automatically GMO-free.

Remember, you're not just "buying food," you're investing in a system, voting, and creating our future. GMOs are not only bad for you, but they're bad for our environment—think soil, air, and water for starters. The only time I make an exception is when I'm shopping at local farmers markets, as some are using all organic practices and non-GMO seed, but have yet to get a certification. This is why knowing your farmers and farm is key. Many people want to buy organic sometimes or just in certain areas, and I understand the transition takes time, but your commitment must be on lock without holes or compromise. We don't pay our bills just sometimes; there are consequences if we don't, right? Don't only care for yourself and your home sometimes. *Be all in.*

You can't wash off DNA. As much as people think washing produce will magically help their non-organic produce, it won't. Consider most of the things on our store shelves. They are not the foods the human body needs. They are "products" that generate revenue for food manufacturers while adding absolutely nothing to the nutritional foundation of consumers.

Here is a thought for you: Is it possible GMOs are making people sick so that Pharma can sell more drugs? Corrupt systems are not just doing things cheap and toxic. We are talking about a criminal cover-up, fraud, and so much more. There is no consequence for those who have committed these crimes. Why is it that people who start to claim there are harmful chemicals in food and talk about the dark side of GMOs (because many praise them), suddenly lose their job or go missing?

How we have not made GMO labeling mandatory by now baffles me. Many GMO companies have spent loads of money fighting this very thing. I wonder why? You, my friend, must be your own advocate and defend your own health. At the same time, we can put pressure on the systems and see reformation.

"Stop counting calories and start counting chemicals."

We live near some fields where there are farm stands, and one day as I was driving home, I noticed a new one had just popped up. I was really excited, as I love local (it reduces carbon footprint, and it's fresh), so I walked up and asked the gal if anything was organic, and she said no. I asked if anything was even non-GMO. Again, no. I told her that was a bummer and went on my way. Within a week, I heard locals rave about this new, local farm stand, talking about how cheap it is and how it's family-run. That part is all great, but y'all, it's toxic! This is why we ask, read labels (not just covers), and never assume.

A study done by UCSF showed 93 percent of people had glyphosate in their system. GMOs are still affecting those of us who eat organic due to surrounding farms. This is why it's essential to follow simple detox protocols, take the right supports for your system, and go "beyond organic."

Not everything organic is healthy, either. I mean, for the love, Doritos has an organic line now. I will celebrate the fact that at least the junk doesn't have pesticides (or does it?), but they're still not the nutrients our body needs. Is it progress? Sure. I far too often see an organic product and then find out it has corn (it's tough to find organic corn) or soy or one of the food enemies listed in this book. Not to mention it will be loaded with organic sugar, which is still a refined sugar and should be totally avoided.

Going beyond organic doesn't just mean avoiding GMOs because there is a lot of organic junk on the market. Organic cookies, candies, bread, and anything you can think of. It's great we are pulling toxins out of food, as it should be, but we still lack the living elements of what our bodies truly crave and need. When we take what God gives us and manipulate it with GMOs and other chemicals, it loses its healing power because it has been altered and life has been taken from it. When it's grown in dead, toxic soil and water, the seed is GMO to the core.

You may think you're making a great choice by choosing fruit, but if it's GMO fruit, don't get too excited. Yes, a conventional piece of fruit is better for you than an organic cookie, and a GMO apple is better than Applebee's, but you truly need to understand how vital organic is. Organic isn't just what's in your food, but how your food is cultivated, grown, and handled. Eating organic is not only safer, but it provides more nutrients for your body. One of the best ways to ensure seed to the soil is pure is by growing your own food. Buying organic (and ideally local) matters beyond our plates; it helps farmers, our waterways, ecosystems, and so much more.

> *"Our food should be our medicine,*
> *and our medicine should be our food."*
> — *Hippocrates*

Allow me to shift gears for a moment as I have to expose more corruption in the food system that some of you may or may not be aware of. Did you know that aborted fetal tissue (HEK 293—human embryonic kidney cells, to be exact) is used to flavor many everyday products? How is this moral, acceptable, or okay? If you needed another reason to eat organically and mindfully, I think this is one.

Some of the companies who use this in their foods are PepsiCo, Kraft Foods, Gatorade, Tazo, Aquafina, Campbell Soup, Solae, Cadbury, and Nestlé. You can also safely assume their products are loaded with GMOs (shocker) and have ties to the system, of course. It's not limited to food products though. The cosmetic and medical industries are also involved.

This part is hard to write, and I can't even fathom it's happening, but companies are selling aborted baby body parts for money. Maybe Planned Parenthood isn't the company most think it is. This is graphic and should upset everyone breathing, and I'm only scratching the surface here. When you read articles that list it all in detail, your mama bear will be fully awake.

Let's consider the current legislation up for passing—it might not be about a woman or a baby, but about a very corrupt system that is much darker than you can imagine. Like I mentioned, fetal parts are being sold for as much as $3,340! There is even a company based out of a major city near me that produces products containing cells from fourteen-week gestation aborted male babies. (To be clear, this type of thing is different than using stem cells for certain treatments.) This is where we are facing immorality, corruption, greed, and far beyond unethical behaviors. This is evil. We must see this new bill overturned and the sanctity of human life upheld.

My personal belief is every life is valuable, has a purpose, and crafted with intention (Jeremiah 1:5). Recently, my eight-year-old daughter and I were talking about this topic as I strongly believe we need to have lots of conversations with our kids (age appropriate) on current issues ranging from sex, human trafficking, abortion, and beyond. She said she felt so sad that these babies won't get to experience all the things in life we do, like family, school, dreams, having a pet (she is an animal lover), and living our dreams. She felt so strongly about it that she wrote a letter to the President. I am very proud of her, and I believe we all need to stop and think like a child at times.

I recognize and acknowledge this is sensitive and controversial. My intention is to share my experience, the truth I know, and the heart I carry. I do not want to trigger or offend, by any means. I know this is tough to read through. I know we all get to believe, decide, act, and live as we choose. I accept, love, and honor right where you are.

> *"A person is a person no matter how small."*
> — *Dr. Seuss*

THE HEALTHCARE SYSTEM

> *"I think we can all agree that conventional medicine does not excel at preventing or reversing chronic disease, which is the biggest challenge we face today."*
> — *Dr. Bradley Kesser*

Where do I even begin with the troubles in our healthcare system? Before we chat about a few, I want to say thank goodness we have healthcare! Although we have systems and issues to tackle and complain about, I am thankful for ER nurses and doctors, surgeons, and first responders. We are a blessed country, despite our current condition and rampant corruption.

We have a few considerable concerns to face when it comes to American healthcare. For starters, Americans pay more for their healthcare; we spend $2.8 trillion on healthcare annually, and that works out to about one-sixth of the total economy and more than $8,500 per person—way more than any other country. At the same time we pay more, we see the doctor less than the universal average. Speaking of expensive (and I am in no way, shape, or form endorsing any medications except using them as legit examples), take the heartburn medication, Nexium. This drug costs $215 in America and $23 in the Netherlands. If you haven't figured this out by now, the "people" making the most money in the medical system are the drug companies.

Now let's get into some more alarming stats. In 1999, the Institute of Medicine (IOM) published a seminal report titled, *To Err Is Human*, which estimated that at least forty-four thousand patients—and as many as ninety-eight thousand—die in hospitals each year as a result of medical errors. A follow-up study published in 2013 argued that the IOM numbers were a vast underestimate and that medical errors contribute to the deaths of between 210,000 and 440,000 patients. On the lower end, that's the equivalent of nearly ten jumbo jets crashing every week—or the entire population of Birmingham, Alabama dying every year.

We spend all of this money on healthcare, yet we still have significant "errors." Interesting. I will also mention the whole insurance situation—Obamacare and Medicare—is a mess. The end.

Aside from the corruption and medical errors (medical errors being the third highest cause of death in America, right behind heart disease and cancer), we have some other concerns within this broken system. This brokenness falls a lot more on insurance companies, lawyers, and farmers than hardworking medical professionals. It isn't the fault of the medical students seeking to do good in the world, giving up years of their life and sleep to only be "educated" from dated materials or a system that says your options are a procedure or prescription. Medical professionals may be in the front, but it's what's going on behind the scenes that tie their hands.

Did you know that the top ten Pharma CEOs are all making over $14 million per year? I'm all about making money. Money isn't bad or wrong, but when that money is tied to corruption, it's an injustice.

> *"Of course, it's tempting to look for the solution and answers in a pill, but let's be real here, when was the last time a pill really fixed your problems or health?"*

Now, I think we are all pretty aware there is a cycle of corruption, dated programs within the industry, and a complete overhaul is needed. The reason we have the numbers we do and such a vast gap doesn't just fall on the system; it also falls on us. How many people get a cold or cough or something simple and go running to the ER or the doctor asking for antibiotics, when that isn't even effective? We are somehow conditioned to think a prescription is a solution. Something as simple as high blood pressure that can be treated through functional medicine is just treated with a pill the conventional way. Where is the investigation and digging to find the cause or root? There isn't. So often we want a quick fix, and don't want to adjust our lifestyle or look at what could be the root of the issue. This does not produce any good results. We also blindly trust that our providers have our best interest in mind, which I'm sorry to say, my friends, they often don't.

"Doctors and insurance companies are treating symptoms, but aren't getting to the root causes."
— *Michael Bernard Beckwith*

I'm going to address why "traditional medicine," or Western healthcare, is dated. Did you know 90 percent of the 3.5 trillion dollars we spend every year goes to treating chronic illnesses? Chronic conditions, such as allergies, autoimmune diseases, digestive issues, hormonal imbalances, and metabolic or neurological problems—which most Americans suffer from daily—are finding solutions in the arena of alternative healthcare, also known as functional medicine. It's funny how we call this practice alternative healthcare when everyone should have "alternative healthcare" so others can choose "Western" or "traditional." Am I right?

I do think both alternative and traditional healthcare have their place though. The most basic way to describe Western healthcare is by the treatment of patients using drugs or surgery. This type of healthcare is treating surface symptoms though, not the root cause. Western healthcare also acts like the brain and body are not connected—huge mistake.

On top of that, it makes it difficult and expensive for people even to have alternative healthcare as an option. In Switzerland, alternative healthcare doctors were able to *change their country's constitution* to have alternative healthcare be the birthright of all Swiss people. Switzerland is the first, and currently only, country where this has happened. Come on, America!

With alternative healthcare, the focus is more on education, prevention (being on the offense), and holistic applications to root causes or symptoms. Even in Western healthcare, a regular practitioner would send you to a specialist, who has the same resources as that doctor: medications and surgeries. Alternative healthcare has over twenty-five options to explore.

Some alternative healthcare options are (but not limited to) herbs, personalized diet plans, answers to in-depth saliva tests, urine tests, and blood work (i.e., allergies, sensitivities, deficiencies), acupuncture, aromatherapy, Ayurveda, chiropractic, cupping, detoxing, herbal medicine, homeopathy, massage, meditation, ozone therapy, therapeutic touch, sound therapy, whole home makeovers (i.e., pantry, medicine cabinets, bathroom cabinets), and yoga. Not only are these safe and effective, but they give more power to the people.

We should be taking more responsibility for our health from our mindsets and emotions to our bodies and beyond. We should not be looking for someone to write us a prescription and send us off to stay in our sick, pain, and victim mindset. Alternative medicine takes a whole-body approach. There could be a great balance of both Western and functional medicine if it were done right. This is also known as *integrative medicine*. I want to give credit to some programs making progress in this area, including Sutter Health and their integrative department.

Integrative medicine shifts the emphasis from establishing what's wrong to finding out how to advance and optimize health, and includes the possibility of personal growth and the goal of transforming your life.

The primary key with health weaved through this entire book is the focus on ownership, action, and *preventative* health. Living a wellness lifestyle is the greatest prevention of disease. It's also personal, which is radically essential when it comes to health. Being treated as a person, versus a chart or number, is a significant step toward better healthcare.

> *"Conventional medicine is the medicine of what.*
> *Functional medicine is the medicine of why."*
> — *Dr. Mark Hyman*

Benefits of Alternative/Functional/Integrative Medicine:
- A focus of diet, lifestyle, and environment
- Addressing the whole person: mind, body, spirit, emotion, heart

- Doctors see the body as it is: an interconnected whole within a larger environment
- Empowering the patient with valuable information, education, tools, and resources
- Getting to the root cause, not just the symptom
- It's about you, not money, a provider, or a system
- It is the future of medicine and healthcare
- Partnering with God's provisions
- Personalized care
- Reversal of disease and chronic
- Science- and evidence-based
- Specialists have extra knowledge, education, and options
- True healthcare and hope for a healthier future

"Conventional medicine isn't really healthcare —it's disease management."

I would highly encourage you to find a functional medicine doctor, and use providers like chiropractors as a regular part of your wellness regime and preventative care. Many doctors even practice online, and with the technology we have available, like email and FaceTime, there are many options for you to look into if you can't find a provider within one or two hours of your location. There is also an amazing doctor treating cancer holistically with wild success rates in Spain, and there is a center in Mexico, as well. These resources are in the back for you.

Together, we can shift our healthcare system with our voices, our choices, and our lifestyles. We need to support our functional medicine community and local practitioners from holistic health coaches, nutritionists, and those trained in functional medicine. Your mind, heart, and body can and will heal when you take the whole-body approach and partner with true healthcare through alternative healthcare options.

THE EDUCATION SYSTEM

Before I dive into this, know not all schools are created equal. Most of the "better" ones are private, Waldorf, or Montessori. I also know there are a lot of teachers and admins pushing for better and for change. We so appreciate and see you. I realize teachers and schools are underpaid and under-resourced, and I want to see a change there, too. I am thankful for schools and all it takes to run them. I don't think all are ill-intentioned.

We should be able to send our kids into schools where teachers care, chemicals are not present, the food isn't just edible but sustainable and healthy, and our kids can learn in small classrooms, free of EMFs and air fresheners. We already have so much to protect our kids from, like bullies, predators, misinformation, propaganda, fear, anxiety, depression, and loneliness. That alone is enough for most parents, never mind worrying about allergies, chemicals, and EMFs.

The other concern in our school system is some of the brainwashing, ten million dittos, overuse of technology, lack of teaching, over-crowded classrooms, medicating "learning disabilities," and pushing mainstream conventional food and medicine onto our kids. Not to mention the mix of beliefs, values, and convictions that may or may not be pushed in the classroom (also known as an agenda), including political ones.

Teachers have told my sons what they think about vaccines, politicians, and "people like me." I have heard far too many stories from customers (students and parents) about what is being said and pushed in many classrooms of all ages, especially colleges. Universities are passing down "Pharma-approved" doctrine, and the medical journals are being sponsored and created by Big Pharma. How is this okay?

Also, how is it alright that one side of the fence is allowed to hate, isolate, bully, and mock, but if the other even speaks the truth, they are kicked out? Double standard much? Parents, please be wise and check your children's curriculum, their teachers' social media pages, and stay involved.

Currently, my boys are both in private school, so we share more of the same values, but not always. Note: *I love my kids' schools* and honor all of their teachers, coaches, staff, and administrators greatly. I am writing a generality of what's happening across the nation, not specific to "my schools." I realize many of you are thinking, "*This is why we homeschool*," and I get that. The reality is that it's not for everyone. I tried it. Twice. I needed a full-on sabbatical after. Many props and praises to the homeschooling families. And much love to the many educators who are bringing love, light, and hope to classrooms. We need you!

THE MEDICAL SYSTEM: PREGNANCY AND BIRTH

I have a theory about all of this. *Brace yourself.* There is a system in place that starts at conception. Let's not act like it's not a coincidence that formula companies send free formula to every pregnant mother. Have you looked at the ingredients in formula? Talk about toxic. It's loaded with sugar and corn! It's at the hospital, then your well-check visits, then in propaganda on your TV shows, newspapers, and magazines. They're conditioning us.

Birth is where a lot of this passion began for me. After my experience with my first son, and even though I had a doula at his hospital birth, I was unaware and uninformed on a lot of things. I wanted a major re-do. I have always loved birth and babies, and encouragement is my middle name, so pairing birth, health, babies, and coaching was a dream. Being in school to be a doula and a health educator affirmed what my gut was trying to tell me: there is a better way.

There was a system in place that was about the money, not my ideal birth. Our bodies are brilliant, and we are strong.

Again, huge disclaimer: not all people working in birth intend to make it sterile over sacred. Not every OB-GYN has a mission to intervene, but a lot do. Did you know that midwives put far more hours into birth and pregnancy practice than OB-GYNs do? They are also equipped to foresee and prevent certain things before they become full-blown issues. Midwives are also known for their bedside manner, support of the birthing woman, baby, breastfeeding, and healthy recovery.

How about inductions? The majority of inductions are not even necessary, but the fact is the moment you have an induction or epidural, your chances for a C-section go up by 50 percent or more. A C-section is far beyond double the price of a natural birth. Interesting, isn't it? Are you connecting the dots?

While we're on the topic of induction, there are things on the market that really shouldn't be in place, and many hospitals have pulled them. Cytotec is one of them. I'm choosing to target this one as it is connected to many complications for babies and moms. If you're a pregnant mom, keep it far, far away. You should also keep vaccines, certain medications, and many toxic personal care and household products far away. I would even go as far as demand to be tested for a gene mutation and allergies before deciding what goes in your body.

NPR did a study and found that only in America the mortality rate is rising in pregnant women. For centuries, we have birthed babies in homes and fields with the assistance of other women. Our bodies and our babies know what to do. We need to trust ourselves. Of course, there can be complications and necessary interventions, but that is rare. The conventional route is preying on vulnerable women, convincing them that their body is broken, the baby is at risk, and they know best. *Lies.* Women are powerful and capable. I have attended many amazing natural births of women who were told they could never have a natural birth. They were right, not in *that* environment. To be surrounded by wise, educated, and intuitive women in your own space or birth center are how things should be, in my opinion, and from my experience.

I had two hospital births and one home birth. I attended many births at every hospital in the Bay Area and Northern California, as well as birth centers and home births. If you want to set yourself and your baby up for the best possible outcome, please get some experts on your team—a chiropractor, midwife, and doula. Studies show women progress much faster at home and shorten labor by over 30 percent when they have a doula and/or midwife.

Now, pregnancy and birth are not all riding on a midwife team. Diet, exercise, environment, and mental health also play a huge role. There are a ton of resources you can connect with if the topic of birth interests you. I'd love to cover all of it, as it is a huge passion and was my practice for over ten years, but this book will turn into a college textbook real quick.

Know that birth is natural, beautiful, sacred, miraculous, magical, and powerful. If you and your baby are healthy, you have no reason to be tied up to machines, a bed, and using medical interventions that are known to delay labor and inhibit natural birth and recovery. Not to mention, your birth experience can affect breastfeeding, bonding, and so much more. In this day and age, we should be seeing significant progress in birth, and it's not moving at the rate it should be for all the information we have access to. My suspicion is the system is involved. I'm going to trust that you will do more digging, or find some amazing midwives, physician assistants, and doulas who can lead you to the light.

THE PERSONAL CARE SYSTEM

Did you know that women use an average of twelve hygiene products each day? Mix that with chemical cleaners (Clorox,

Pine-Sol, and Windex, to name a few), and we wonder why we have a headache or "don't feel right." These products have known carcinogens in them, not to mention pesticides and hormone and reproductive disruptors. Decades of studies indicate serious health issues (including, but not limited to asthma, cancer, and infertility) are on the rise, and are due in some part to our ongoing exposure to toxic chemicals—whether it's in the shower, on our commute, while we eat lunch at a local restaurant, or when we clean our kitchens at home.

> *"Before you ask why non-toxic cleaning*
> *and body products are so expensive,*
> *ask why the others are so cheap."*
> — *Catie Gett*

There are tens of thousands of unsafe chemicals in the market today, especially in the skincare and beauty industry. You read that right: *tens of thousands,* and America barely regulates the ingredients allowed in our products. The FDA has only banned about *thirty* chemicals, where Europe has banned nearly fourteen hundred ingredients and chemicals. Shocking, I know!

Feel free to grab your beauty and cleaning products and give them a scan on EWG or look up their ingredients—scary stuff. As I mentioned, what many other countries ban is entirely acceptable here, and we wonder why our disease rates, death rates, and allergy rates are skyrocketing. I'm attempting to leave no stone unturned here, friends. How about those "air fresheners" in your car and home and plug-ins (more like chemical shiz-storms)? For clarity sake, shiz is how Christian hippies say the s-word. You're welcome. We also say *bless it* instead of other phrases. You're very welcome.

There was a study done in 2008 (imagine what we can find in 2019), proving that the leading brands in cleaning products and air fresheners emitted large amounts of chemicals. The kicker though? All the products tested in this study emitted at least one chemical that would be considered toxic and hazardous under federal laws, but they were not on the product's label. Some of the chemicals they found are known as the active ingredients found in paint thinner and nail-polish remover. *Umm, what?* But you want to know if essential oils are safe?

Now, let's talk *fragrance* (in cleaning products, candles, cosmetics, laundry products, personal products, and air fresheners). Do you notice when you read the back of your lotion bottle, glass cleaner, or fabric softener that you can read the ingredient "fragrance," but there's no additional information about what that fragrance is made from? The Federal Fair Packaging and Labeling Act of 1973 require cosmetic companies to label all the ingredients on their products, except fragrance. I'm not exaggerating when I say that the term "fragrance" can be anything, and it's more often times than not found to be carcinogenic, as well as petroleum-based. (If you aren't aware, gasoline is derived from this same petroleum ingredient.) This book would get far too long if I give you any more facts, stats, and studies on fragrance. I think you're getting it.

Earlier, I mentioned that even soy candles are garbage. Let me explain. Burning a soy candle will release small amounts of the carcinogens and toxins found in paraffin wax. This is because most soy candles on the market are not even 100 percent soy, so they contain a high percentage of this poisonous paraffin wax. They're also mostly made up of fragrances and dyes, and even if they are essential oil-based, you're still dealing with soy and paraffin. Also, essential oils are not meant to be mixed and burned, as it changes their molecules. Beeswax candles are an upgraded choice for all my candle-lovers out there. However, many beeswax candles on the market are only 51 percent beeswax, so be sure you see 100 percent beeswax on the label. If you can't afford beeswax candles, your options are to make your own, go candle-free, or use aromatherapy instead. Soy has zero benefits on every level, and it's GMO (91 percent of soy is). Basically, you're supporting GMOs when you buy soy candles. We know soy is harmful to the environment as well, where beeswax actually reduces allergies and asthma.

This next one might fall under the TMI arena (not for those of us who work in the birth field), but did you know women's hygiene products are full of chemicals, too, unless they are certified organic? Just an FYI, I'm partial to a DivaCup. We can talk about that in person. I'm sure many of you are now googling DivaCup—have fun with that!

Tampons (specifically the non-organic ones) contain that nasty carcinogen, glyphosate. Anything we put inside our bodies—yes, especially down there—gets easily absorbed into our mucous membrane, and then into our bloodstream where it becomes toxic to our body. When we repeatedly expose our bodies to these toxins, we undoubtedly are going to increase our risk of infertility, endometriosis, and thyroid disorders, not to mention cancer.

Personal care products do not just affect women, to be very clear. Men are just as exposed to and use toxic, chemical-filled deodorants, cologne, toothpaste, lotions, shaving creams, and the like.

> *"In America, we call it lobbying. Everywhere*
> *else it's called bribery and corruption."*
> — *Unknown*

THE CURRENT CLIMATE

Did you know we are currently at a thirty-year low for birth rates? The lowest year for births in thirty years was in 2017. I want to connect that to our unhealthy and very toxic systems, as well as some culture shifts, and this will get dicey. I want to touch on the subject of abortion. According to Lila Rose, forty-one million babies died before birth in 2018. Abortion is the leading cause of death in America. As much as rates have gone down in some areas, it's still a widespread issue. Yes, I am pro-life. We can still be friends if you're not, zero judgment. If you have had an abortion, I love you, and I hope you'll hear my heart in this section.

I know it's hard to hear and handle, and I need to bring up more: autism, mental health, and learning disabilities. Now, I'm not going into it, but I'm bringing it up in regard to chemicals, systems, and birth statistics. Vaccines Revealed and Dr. Stephanie Seneff have a statistic that one in two boys will be on the autism spectrum by 2025! *This is crazy!*

I do believe ultrasounds, gut biome, mold, genome, vaccines, EMFs, environmental toxins, medications, food, and household chemicals (I talk more about these things in the next chapter) are all connected to autism. The amount, how, and why? I'm not sure. I know many people who are treating and reversing it with diet, detox, CBD, and a non-toxic home. Specifically, one of my favorite health gurus I send people to is *Medical Medium* and all of Anthony William's books. *Liver Rescue*, also by William, is a must-read for anyone with an autoimmune disease, autism, or metal-toxicity. As with anything, *there is always hope.*

There is an epidemic that Dr. Mark Hyman talks about, called broken brain. "Broken brain" is Dr. Mark Hyman's term, and he has a documentary and podcast on it, but we will change it up and talk about the deeper root. The deeper root here is the whole idea how "food makes your mood," and how silent enemies are not being addressed in connection to mental health issues (i.e., mold, EMFs, gene mutations, mercury and metal poisoning, pesticide poisoning, gut health). Broken brain affects one in eight children, one in four adults, and one in two elderly. To do more research on this topic, I recommend checking out Dr. Hyman's documentary I've referenced for you in the back.

Back to "the systems." (Wow, I've never said "systems" this much in my life.) They do not have our best interest in mind.

Sadly, their interest is in their success, shortcuts, and their bottom line, not in ethical values, sustainability, or care. Most don't even know what fair trade or ethical means. Of course, there are exceptions where some companies might not be healthy or wholesome, but maybe they are doing their best, and they don't know better. I don't believe every company is purely evil, but I will be honest with you—many are.

If you don't believe that's possible, watch the movie, *Erin Brockovich*. This kind of madness is happening every single day. Don't get me started on cell towers and what those are doing to our health and communities. There is more on that to come. It's completely unacceptable the things they do not tell us (let that sink in for a moment), the things they hide from us, and the ways they've entirely deceived us.

PROFITS OVER PATIENTS

Unfortunately, every arm of the system is in it for themselves. Now, I don't think every one of these corporations or those who work for them truly understand the damage. I believe they think they are doing good in some way, but there are still companies who know the truth, yet continue to produce harmful foods or harmful products. Let's not act like politicians aren't pushing bills for profit. There are far too many examples of this.

> *"We won't have a cure for disease*
> *until we first have a cure for greed."*
> — *Dr. Sachin Patel*

Did you know the household name, Johnson & Johnson, has been the number one baby hygiene brand for over twenty years? All along, they knew there were cancer-causing chemicals in their products, but it wasn't until 2015 and into 2018 that these facts started circulating and a lawsuit was against them.

Even still, with all the information out there and easily accessible, people continue not just to buy Johnson & Johnson but to sell Johnson & Johnson. How is this okay? Going back to the cycle, Johnson & Johnson offers samples in the hospital. Johnson & Johnson and Pampers make the cute commercials. Remember, the devil doesn't always look scary! It's all part of training our brain to accept and *trust without question.*

Besides the companies who are obvious with their chemicals and corruption, the ones who tick me off the most are the ones who greenwash. The ones who put the farm on the front and say "all natural," but when you look at the ingredients, you find nothing natural about it at all.

It's the same with the gluten-free companies who label many things "gluten-free" now, but they've always been gluten-free (like water or beef jerky). They are labeling their products "gluten-free" as a marketing ploy to get those who don't understand to think it's healthy. In reality, there is corn, sugar, and GMOs loaded into these products!

The same goes for "vegan." "Vegan" does not mean healthy. You could have a vegan donut that's full of white sugar, white flour, and corn. All of which are incredibly inflammatory and immune-suppressing. Yet, products can be labeled "vegan," which many people translate as "healthy." This is the system I'm talking about—it does not have your best interest in mind! These companies are selling a product only to make a profit. As I mentioned, I'm all about making money, but can we do it the right way, for the love?

"It's time to protect people, not corporate profits."

Selling products and doing business the "right way" should be the primary goal of every health company. They should want to make a good product, do things ethically, morally, and sustainably, and they should want to make a difference on the earth and in their communities. Of course, they want to make a profit, which is great, and I fully support that. I have one of those companies. Money is not the root of all evil. Money isn't the issue; the heart is. The question isn't *Do you have money?* the question is *Does money have you?*

YOU VOTE WITH YOUR DOLLARS

When you buy from a specific store or a particular brand, you are voting for them and what they believe. My family has made a personal choice not to support brands or products that do not do things with integrity, honesty, sustainability, and ethics. Where and how we spend our money says what we believe and what we support. I will not support a system that is causing sickness, stress, addiction, or anything other than your best self. Will you join me on this mission?

Yes, the health element greatly matters to me, but there is also a principle in place for me when it comes to the products and companies I choose to support. The meat industry is one for starters. Before learning about my blood type, I was a vegetarian for seven years. I also learned about sustainable, regenerative farming and the fact that there are actually "happy cows" and truly grass-fed, grass-finished, and sustainable methods of farming. Regenerative farming is a whole book in itself (actually it is, *Kiss the Ground*, by Josh Tickell). If we do not change the way we are currently farming, our entire earth is at risk. If you're vegan, you might think you are helping the earth, but I want you to know that the production of corn, soy, and wheat is harming our earth as well. I highly recommend grabbing a copy of *Kiss the Ground* and following them, along with Be Love Farm, to understand the importance of regenerative farming.

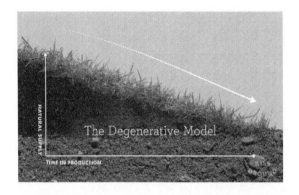

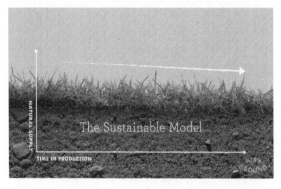

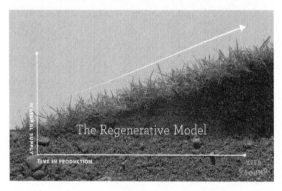

In a nutshell, regenerative farming is the way crops and animals were originally designed to grow and to thrive. Having animals and crops co-mingle to co-benefit is the way it should be.

Perfectly done rows are the exact opposite of regenerative.

Regenerative farming is a whole new arena just starting to be addressed more and more. People are beginning to realize this type of farming is vital to the future of our cities and for our children. If you've seen *Bee Movie,* you know what I mean, and that's just one example. Do you realize all these pesticides and herbicides being sprayed go into our water systems and our surrounding communities, and they are harming the pollinators that we need?

Systems are not just our choices, homes, and the way we grow our food; more corruption is happening all around us. In our kids' schools. In hospitals. Big-box stores. Your kids' favorite cartoon shows. Take note of the sponsors all over the subways and bus stops.

On top of all this, it's proven that companies are targeting minority communities with their junk and ads, as well as making bad choices easier while good choices are out of sight and not promoted. Why is it that every single store has candy and chips at the register now, including Staples and Old Navy? It wasn't like this just a few years ago.

It blows my mind to see what schools are serving at lunch, as well as what's handed out at sports camps and events. It doesn't even go together or makes sense. The same goes for hospital visits. Why in the world are we giving sick or recovering patients food and drinks that suppress their immune system and cause health issues?

The simplest explanation to this would be that it's all part of one corrupt system. Or maybe just a system that, over the years, slowly began to compromise in the name of science, GMOs, saving a dollar, and convenience. The corruption goes as far as brand-recognition and knowing the consumer will trust them just because their brand is familiar. Can I expose something for you? Just because the front is labeled "nutritional" doesn't mean there is actual nutrition inside. I know some of this is hard to believe, comprehend, and understand. Feel free to pause and take a moment. Please do your research, and I encourage you to keep reading.

If you're skeptical that there is foul play, how does it sit with you? I've read reports saying there are heavy metals, such as arsenic and lead, in forty-five packaged fruit juices. *What?* Things like this are happening daily. What is in, on, and around our "food" is unacceptable. The craziest part is the Centers for Disease Control and Prevention (CDC) doesn't recommend an overhaul of the system or demand the companies to change how they make the juice. Their recommendation is for parents to give less of it to their kids. There are reports after reports like this regarding food, yet we carry on and rebuy without thinking twice. What food companies and the CDC are calling "safe" means something completely different to you and me. Their version of "safe" still means poisonous, toxic, and harmful. Buyer beware.

"A patient cured is a customer lost."

It would be so much easier to believe all these companies are looking out for us and want us to be healthy, right? Let's get real, do you think these companies want you to know you could drink a cup of green tea, use some essential oils, and avoid sugar and gluten for a few days versus paying for a doctor visit to get some medication? I mean how many medication commercials do we actually have? How about magazines and newspapers? It's ridiculous. Do you see any commercials promoting holistic wellness? Do you see any big brands promoting alternative medicine? Interesting assessment, isn't it?

Even more interesting is the connection between presidents, boards, and positions within certain companies like the FDA, Big Food, and Big Pharma. I think they are trusting that we're just asleep at the wheel so we don't notice. It is in our best interest to be educated and informed so we can make our own decisions and advocate for ourselves, whether we are at the grocery store or the hospital.

Again, as I've stated many times in this book, I am not against the medical system, but I am against corruption and deception. This is not a knock on highly-educated medical professionals. I believe most of them do not know better. Many doctors have said they did not receive any training or information on many of the things addressed. Thank God for surgeons, first responders, nurses, and doctors who live with conviction and compassion. I have so much respect for those who are there in crisis and at bedsides.

I am also not one to sit back and see people being misled and misguided, to have them harm their health and say, "Oh well! Not my problem." Turning a blind eye isn't my organic jam. I am one of those people who take personal responsibility for my community as much as possible. We need to have the mentality of *we* versus *me* more often. I know it can be scary to stand up for truth, what's right, and what you believe in, but what is even more terrifying to me would be to sit back and do nothing, when I know I could have done *something*. It's in my nature (shout-out to all the Eights on the Enneagram) to lead, teach, share, and empower.

> **"If the system of Western medicine was really dedicated to people's health, then pharmaceutical companies would be celebrating when drug sales dropped."**
> — *Peter Crone*

Let's address (more like tip-toe around) the pharmaceutical crisis and opioid epidemic. This is sensitive and risky, I know. As stated more times than I can count, if something has more side effects than benefits, why are we blindly trusting it? (Counting is hard, guys. Math is not my fave. All hail the numbers people in the world!) People say you should judge a doctor by how many medications they get you off, not on. I am not an expert by any means; certain things are more common sense than needing a Ph.D. We have to get honest and realize Big Pharma isn't having meetings about our wellbeing. If they are, let me know. I'd love to be there. In 2018 alone, there were one hundred and twenty-six new prescription drugs on the market. What the actual? One in ten people over the age of twelve are on something.

One of the craziest things to me is when I have a customer or friend trust what a doctor says, having done no research whatsoever, but when I suggest they drink celery juice, try CBD, take vitamin C, or consider alternative options, they respond with *Is that safe?* or *Let me check with my doctor first.* Listen, Virginia, I don't think that aspartame in your gum is safe, but you're chewing it. I don't think that a prescription drug with the possible side effects of death, blindness, or a coma is safe, yet you take it. I don't think that perfume you spray every day is good for the environment or your hormones, but spray away. By all means, please consult WebMD and your doctor about some zinc.

I don't have the solution, remedy, or potion (religious people, settle down) for this crisis, but I can't not talk about it in a wellness book. The effects of prescription drugs are not limited to addiction, overdosing, scarring of neural pathways, emotional numbness, suicide, digestive issues, sleep issues, and so much more. It's no secret that some of these Pharma companies have a mission to get you from the cradle to the grave with their "products." Did you know America has 5 percent of the world's population, yet we are consuming 80 percent of the world's opiates? America is hurting big time.

When we are numbing ourselves, getting high, damaging our livers, or suffering, we aren't getting the highest essence of our true selves, and that fact *scares me.* We're not able to focus, achieve, heal, or deal at a "normal" level due to side effects. It's messier than a two-year-old with an ice cream cone out here, y'all.

Yes, awareness and slow changes are happening, but not at

the rate we need. Over seventy thousand people died from an overdose in 2017 alone, and those are only the reported ones. The pain people are in is very real, and the opioid crisis is real. The corruption within the whole wheel is deep and dark, and we must shine light, speak truth, and do better.

HOW TO WIN IN A CORRUPT WORLD

> *"Let us not be a society of people who clean up the outside of us, but not the inside."*
> — *Darleen Santore*

The good news is the less is more in the non-toxic world. You save money in this area so you can apply that to your organic food and supplement budget instead. *Winning*.

Here are some simple things you can do right now:
- Choose wisely and make slow changes.
- Donate to people in the trenches of this mission.
- Email your city officials and senators. Let's get chemicals removed from our schools and parks. Say *no* to Roundup!
- Make your own cleaners and detergents, or buy upgraded versions. Remember, we are replacing and upgrading, not just removing.
- Read the connected articles and know the things to avoid listed in *Enemies of Health*.
- Research your brands.
- Scan and search items on EWG.
- Share this knowledge with three people.
- Shop local.

I hope this chapter has been an awakening for you to see these systems around us that should be "supporting us" are not for us at all. Many of these things were never even created for our consumption, and sadly most of them are numbing us and dumbing us down. They are destroying our bodies, minds, and spirits, along with our quality of life, relationships, and purpose. It doesn't have to be this way. There is a better, elevated, and upgraded way, my friends. It's healing through wisdom.

I will not go on an environmental rant here because we have covered *a lot*. At the end of the day, these chemicals are not good for us. They are not good for our planet, our ecosystems, animals, air, water, *all of it*. From plastics and narcotics to pesticides and the many other chemicals we talked about, it's all no bueno. *Not just for our mind, body, and spirit, but the earth we live.*

We must fight for transparency and change. We must fight for sustainability and fewer chemicals. We must fight for our health. Let's be the change. Let's do this for something bigger than ourselves. *It is our watch.* We must take action and not settle. Yes, knowledge is power, but knowledge without action doesn't help anyone. I charge you to be a person of change, action, and intention.

As much as I feel pretty woke, non-toxic, and your go-to neighborhood medicine woman, I'm still with you on this journey. People in my house sometimes buy things with their own money. I once found a stick of Degree on my son's desk, and he said I acted like it was drugs. True story. (For the record, Schmidt's and Every Man Jack are products we buy for our teen boys. Bless it.) You will find there are non-toxic options in every area we've covered from salons, medication, and household items. There is always an upgraded option.

If we have all of these articles, documentaries, apps, labels, and YouTube videos, why do we choose to watch another episode of *The Bachelor* instead of getting informed and "arming" ourselves? We've lifted the veil. We've pulled the curtain back. However you see it, here we are. Your health, your home's health, and your future health are dependent on your upgraded choices because it truly matters. You are here reading this right now at the right time. No, it's not too late. The time is now. You are here because you care, and you will be a voice. Make a new choice and live your best life. I believe this to be true, and know *I am in the fight with you.*

CHAPTER FIVE

ENEMIES OF HEALTH

THE THINGS NOBODY WANTS TO TALK ABOUT

"The greatest wealth is health."
— Virgil

In the spirit of being brave and confrontational, yet compassionate, I'd like to talk about the things no one else does, and if they do, they are banned, blackmailed, sometimes killed (pray for me), mocked, and criticized. *Gulp.* By no means do I know it all, have a complete list, or the exact answers. I'm focused here on giving you some things to think about and look for on your labels so you can protect yourself, your home, and your family from harm.

To give you a taste of how important this is to talk about, a report done by Columbia University's School of Public Health estimated that diet and environmental activity caused 95 percent of cancer cases. Also, almost one and a half million people are diagnosed with cancer each year. There are seventeen million new cases of cancer worldwide, and close to ten million deaths from cancer worldwide.

> *"Just because something is common doesn't*
> *mean it is normal. Cancer is common,*
> *but it's not normal."*
> — *Kris Vallotton*

In the previous chapter, I told you about things that mainstream systems will not address, and now I'm going to touch on some sensitive subjects that will require you to do research on your own and come to your own conclusions. Through my years of research, studying, and becoming more aware and involved day-to-day, here are some things I found shocking and disturbing that affect our health, even if we're doing all the right things and using all organic products.

Enemies Out of Our Control:
Air Pollution
Chemtrails — *geoengineering and surrounding pesticide crops*
Chemotherapy
EMFs — *electromagnetic fields from laptops, TVs, tablets, wearables, phones, and cell towers, especially 5G. Run if you have one near you!*
Environmental toxins — *not limited to, but coming from plants, refineries, oil spills, litter, fire retardants, toxic farming, and smog*
Fragrance — *found in cleaning products, personal care products, stores, public restrooms, and gyms*
Roundup — *please look up the Monsanto school district lawsuit*
Unnecessary surgeries and procedures — *or standard, basic procedures gone wrong*
Water — *the amount of narcotics, fire retardants, pesticides, and metals in our tap water is insane. This is why we use a Berkey filter, and if we must buy bottled, it's Essentia brand.*

I can't skip over this part without addressing how toxic fluoride is. Buckle up and have your phone ready to send a shiz storm to your people with all the mind-blown emojis. For starters, fluoride is a neurotoxin. It's a harmful substance that calcifies the pineal gland, disrupts your thyroid, blood sugar levels, and lowers your IQ. It is also connected to Alzheimer's disease, and it was used in concentration camps. *Yes,* I'm serious. Rock phosphate (a type of fluoride) was used during the Cold War period for the extraction of uranium to make bombs.

Fluoride is poison and covered up in the name of "dental health." Fluoride is more toxic than lead, but slightly less toxic than arsenic. This is why it has long been used in rodenticides and pesticides to kill pests, like rats and insects. The main fluoride chemical added to water today is hydrofluorosilicic acid, an industrial byproduct from the phosphate fertilizer industry. It attaches to aluminum, which already occurs in our water supply, and it can pass through the blood-brain barrier and kill brain cells. Fluoride is so toxic it is considered hazardous waste by the EPA. Why is it legal for fluoride to be in our drinking water and toothpaste when it's illegal to dump fluoride into our lakes and rivers?

Surveys show there are significantly fewer people with cancer and cavities when water supplies are not fluoridated. Another reason I choose not to buy any bottled water other than Essentia brand is because even if the bottled water says it's filtered, it usually has fluoride in it. This also includes fruit juices from concentrate; they are reconstituted with fluoridated water.

Did you know a tube of toothpaste with fluoride can kill a child under the age of six? Um, not safe. I know you're thinking, *"But we don't eat our toothpaste."* Even if you don't swallow your toothpaste, unhealthy levels of fluoride are still absorbed sublingually through the capillaries under your tongue and go directly into your bloodstream. You know how a lot of homeopathic meds and herbs call for holding under your tongue? (I.e., CBD, colloidal silver, etc.) Yeah, it matters. Why would we want to use this substance for consumption by humans? I mean, all in the name of "dental health," yet it does nothing to benefit our teeth. Other countries don't need this "miracle for their teeth!" Again, America, *why?*

This certainly is a book in itself, so I suggest you watch some documentaries, find a fluoride-free dentist, and switch all your fluoride-containing products as soon as possible. Two great documentaries you can watch free online are *An Inconvenient Tooth* (best name ever) and *Fluoridegate: An American Tragedy*. This is one of the most simple and affordable things you can do for your health right now.

On the flip side of all of these enemies outside of our control are things within our control. However, people have told us these things will help us or that they are good for us. I have listed them here, but not in full. I'm pulling out the top ones, and some that are not as well-known as others so you can be on alert!

The majority of food additives invented in the last few decades have been created for the sole purpose to improve the bottom line of the food industry—not our health. Now, to be clear, you may or may not be affected by one or more of these. Some you will know off the bat, and some will take some digging. Often our human reasoning wants one particular thing to blame and train to ride, but health isn't as simple as that. There are many levels and layers to complete wholeness, so please take it with a grain of Himalayan pink salt.

<u>**Enemies Within Our Control:**</u>
Alcohol
Drugs
GMOs — *genetically modified organisms*
Implants and self-improvement procedures — *keep reading for more information on implant poisoning, tattoos, and mold*
Mindsets and heartsets — *see* Mindfulness, Meditation, and Mindsets

Tobacco
Top ten worst ingredients in processed food:
1. Bad oils and shortenings
2. White flour and sugar
3. High-fructose corn syrup
4. Artificial sweeteners
5. Sodium benzoate and potassium benzoate
6. Butylated hydroxyanisole (BHA)
7. Sodium nitrates and sodium nitrites
8. Blue, Green, Red, and Yellow food coloring
9. MSG and BHT
10. Artificial flavors, TBHQ, and lupin (a legume)

Vaping

"More people are dying from drive-thru's than drive-by's."

Enemies in Food:
Aspartame — *also called AminoSweet, NutraSweet, Equal Spoonful, Sweet'N Low, Canderel, Benevia, E951 (U.K. & European Code)*
Baking powder
Canola oil — *rapeseed oil*
Caramel color
Cellulose
Citric acid
Cobalamin — *vitamin B12*
Colorose
Condensed milk
Confectioners sugar
Corn flour
Corn masa
Cornmeal
Corn oil

Corn sugar
Corn syrup
Cornstarch
Cottonseed oil
Cyclodextrin
Cysteine
Dextrin
Dextrose
Diacetyl
Diglyceride
Erythritol
Food starch
Fructose — *any form*
Glucose
Glutamate
Glutamic acid
Glycerides
Glycerin
Glycerol
Glycerol monooleate
Glycine
Hemicellulose
High-fructose corn syrup
Hydrogenated starch
Hydrolyzed vegetable protein
Inositol
Inverse syrup
Inversol
Invert sugar
Isoflavones
Lactic acid
Lecithin
Leucine
Lysine

Maltodextrin
Maltose
Mannitol
Methylcellulose
Milk powder
Milo starch
Modified starch
Mono and diglycerides
Monosodium glutamate *(MSG)*
Oleic acid
Phenylalanine
Phytic acid
Protein isolate
Shoyu
Sorbitol
Soy flour
Soy isolates
Soy lecithin
Soy milk
Soy oil
Soy protein
Soy sauce
Starch
Stearic acid
Sugar
Tamari
Tempeh
Teriyaki marinades
Textured vegetable protein
Threonine
Tocopherols — *vitamin E*
Tofu
Trehalose
Triglyceride

Maltitol	**Vegetable fat**
Malt	**Vegetable oil**
Malt syrup	**Whey** — *unless organic grass-fed*
Malt extract	**Xanthan gum** — *not always bad depending on company source*

Additional Enemies:

Asbestos

Aluminum foil — *yes, it's a toxin and heavy metal*

Antibiotic consumption

Beauty and personal care products — *sunblock and bug spray are two of the most toxic*

BVO — *brominated vegetable oil. A flame retardant found in many drinks such as, but not limited to:*

> **Ensure** — *a drink suggested by doctors*

> **Glucola** — *a glucose test that contains tons of toxins*

Carrageenan — *a popular ingredient in lots of organic things. Beware though, it may be organic from other countries, but it is sprayed to enter the U.S.*

Chlorine

Chromium-6

Dental treatments and poor oral health — *such as root canals and metal fillings, plus all the fluoride.*

Dioxins

Energy drinks

Furniture and mattresses — *most are made with toxins, sprayed, leak toxins into your home (i.e., fungicides, fire retardants)*

Gas pumps — *another one that falls into air issues*

Gene mutations — *MTHFR and COMT*

Heavy metals — *including aluminum, lithium, mercury, arsenic*

Household products — *cleaning, yard, paint, pest control, EMFs, LED lights, the air*

Microwaves — *more EMFs*

Mold and mildew

Nail salons and hair salons — *toxic ingredients such as solvents, plasticizers, acids, and resins are commonly found in nail care products. (Studies from the Northern California Cancer Center and Asian Health Services of Oakland show that the women who work in these nail salons suffer acute health effects from the chemicals that they work with each day.)*

New clothes — *typically covered in chemicals from the journey overseas*

Non-fat and soy products — *the 'bad wrap' on 'fats.' These types of products are labeled and pushed as health foods.*

Old-school food pyramid — *SAD diet*

Pesticides

Phthalates

Plastics and BPA — *bisphenol A*

Polychlorinated biphenyl

Prescription meds/narcotics/birth control — *see* The System is Not Your Friend

SLS — *sodium lauryl sulfate*

Soda — *including and especially diet soda*

Sports drinks

Tap water and fluoride

Toxic cookware — *especially Teflon, plastic, and scratched cookware (cast iron and stainless are best)*

Underwire bras — *EMF magnets*

Vaccines — *please don't jump ship here*

X-ray machines/MRIs — *more EMFs*

"Eighty-five percent of disease is environmental."

Effects of Environmental Toxins:
Allergies and asthma
Altered metabolism
Cancer
Chronic viral infections
Depressed immune system

Endocrine disorders
Enzyme dysfunction
Fatigue
Headaches
Hormonal imbalances
Lower ability to tolerate or handle stress
Muscle and vision problems
Neurological disorders
Nutritional deficiencies
Obesity
Reproductive disorders

> *"Chronic disease is a foodborne illness.*
> *We ate our way into this mess,*
> *and we must eat our way out."*
> — *Dr. Mark Hyman*

Enemies People Are Not Addressing or Aware Of:

Adrenaline — *in excess*

Autoimmune diseases and chronic illnesses — *Lyme, candida, multiple sclerosis, rheumatoid arthritis, lupus, celiac disease, anemia, vitiligo, psoriasis, and type-one diabetes. Sixty percent of America suffers from chronic diseases, and one in six people have an autoimmune disease.*

Cortisol levels

Dangers of overusing antibiotics

Deficiencies — *magnesium, iodine, vitamin B, iron, testosterone (especially in men over 35), and D3*

Digestive issues — *small intestine bacterial overgrowth (SIBO)*

Dopamine — *addiction*

Dormant viruses or bacteria

Gut health, liver health, and parasites

Healthy hormones — *estrogen dominance, adrenal, and thyroid health. This doesn't just affect women.*

Histamine
Lack of genome and epigenetic understanding
Melatonin
Mindsets — *toxic thinking and speaking is a real enemy*
Misdiagnoses — *including false positives or diagnoses, and covering up or missing allergies, sensitivities, and reactions*
Mitochondria disease and unbalance
Serotonin levels
Toxic stress — *not all stress is bad*

SILENT ENEMIES AROUND US: AIR

The next few enemies we will cover are silent, which make them tricky. The first chat is going to be about air. Yep, I know it now feels like we should all live in a bubble. I get that. Who is joining me to live in a yurt on an organic farm on a mountain top? *Just kidding.* We won't have to because we have tools, resources, and amazing things to help us! Fear not, yet be wise.

Even in 2019, we still have poor air quality issues not just outdoors, but indoors. Everything from volatile organic compounds (VOCs), pet dander, harmful gases, mold, allergens, formaldehyde, dust mites, chemicals, and viruses. Even in a non-toxic home, you are still exposed to these air pollutants indoors, especially in commercial buildings. Thankfully, there are things we can do to ensure our home air quality is pure, healthy, and adding value to our daily lives.

<u>Ensuring Your Air Quality:</u>
Air purifiers — *Austin Air or AIR Doctor*
Bamboo charcoal blocks
Beeswax candles
Change air filters often
Essential oil diffusers

Open windows
Plants — *snake plants, rubber plant, Boston ferns, and bamboo palms*
Salt lamps

> *"If your health isn't in alignment, nothing is."*
> — *Preston Smiles*

SILENT ENEMIES AROUND US: MOLD

The other thing you will want to investigate in your home is mold. It's crazy what mold will do to your health, and not enough people are talking about it or evaluating if it's the missing link to their health issues. It's not just in older homes or in cases of flooding, but even leaks can lead to black mold. I have three friends who were significantly affected by unknown mold in their homes. They had chronic colds, coughs, pain, and unexplainable symptoms, even though they were living and eating non-toxic. Mold is not a joke or something you mess around with.

It's a fact that 22 percent of homes or buildings have some mold. Mold releases spores as it feeds on organic materials in common household materials like drywall, carpet, insulation, or subfloors exposed to moisture. It could be from a leak, flood, or even overwatering gardens and standing water. These spores, if ingested or inhaled, can cause a range of unpleasant and dangerous symptoms in all ages. It's far more common and toxic than people realize.

Mold isn't just toxic; it can lead to mold-poisoning. It has a long history of being an enemy of bacteria, and absolutely toxic to your mitochondria. Those antibiotics you take that kill bacteria? They come from mold!

Mold lowers your liver's immune system (the liver is considered your third brain). The real issue with mold is for those who have compromised immune systems, dormant viruses, or chronic illness. It is adding a more massive load to an already-taxed system. This is why mold affects everyone differently, and to be clear, it affects everyone negatively. Everyone reacts and responds differently, as we all have different biology and brains (i.e., liver, colon, gut).

Fungicides are also a cause of mold in food. We see a rise in these issues and bacteria because mold is becoming fungicide-resistant. They are found all over new furniture, new clothes, and in toxic air fresheners. Even if you don't have them at home, they are in many public restrooms.

Most coffee has mold (mycotoxins), too. This is why you should make sure you're brewing "mold-free" organic, fair trade beans. Buying this type of coffee is not just a good idea, but a must. It's not only in the beans, but mold can be trapped in coffee pots and Keurigs, too. This is why I suggest making coffee with a French press or pour over to avoid mold.

<u>Symptoms of Toxic Mold:</u>
Abdominal pain and new Crohn's disease
Allergy-like symptoms
Chronic sinus infections or strep throat
Excessively stiff joints and muscle pain
Extremely poor memory
Frequent nosebleeds and unexplained bruising
Hashimoto's thyroiditis
Headaches
Incredible thirst
Intense need to urinate without a full bladder
Joint pain
Lightheadedness and vertigo
Metallic taste in the mouth
Mood swings
Muscle weakness

New food allergies — *especially to gluten and dairy*
Rashes
Repeat miscarriages
Rheumatoid arthritis and gout
Sudden change in electrostatic discharge when you touch things
Tingling feelings and restless legs
Unexplained, repeated coughs and colds — *especially at night*
Weight gain
Worsening of nearly every neurodegenerative and autoimmune disease

You should always test a new space for mold and any time after a leak, seeing constant standing water, and spots on walls, floors, or ceilings. I experienced mold sickness, and who knows if it's all out of my system. I had mold on my bathroom walls from the age of thirteen to eighteen. My bathroom growing up was carpeted and didn't have a window or vent. My mom would bleach it or have us clean it with Simple Green (just wow). Horrible, right?

I have other friends who had to sell their newly-purchased home due to hidden mold, and they found out only after experiencing mold symptoms. One girlfriend of mine thought she was in the clear because they had their home tested, but forgot to check the attic. Mold is no joke, friends. It isn't something you bleach out or ignore. Testing your home is one step. The next is testing your body. A GENIE test would be a great place to start.

Signs of Mold:
Discolored wood or walls
Leaking pipes
Musty smell
Trouble concentrating
Unexplained fatigue
Water damage, soft/wet walls, bubbling paint

<u>**Common Places to Check For Mold:**</u>
Attics, garages, basements, or subfloors — *commonly missed and are mold hot spots*
Bathtub or shower caulking
Dishwashers
Toilet tanks
Under the bathroom and kitchen sink
Window sills — *sometimes collect condensation in the winter, which causes mold to grow*

If you have been exposed to mold or suspect mold-poisoning:
1. Take Dr. Ann Shippy's mold test.
2. Get a test kit from CitriSafe. It's affordable and comes with a free consultation once your mold report is complete. They also carry a non-toxic mold killing solution that works.
3. *Bio-Balance Now* carries a fogger with a non-toxic solution that works exceptionally well.
4. Remove and eradicate, ideally professionally. If you are still having symptoms after a home detox, it's possible you're dealing with a virus, bacteria, or underlying "illness" of some type which you will want to explore, treat, and heal.
5. Detox and remove mold from your body (this process can take thirty days to six months depending on your immune system) with:
   - Activated Charcoal (internal)
   - Bentonite clay (internal)
   - Certain essential oils from doTERRA: oregano, On Guard, lime, rosemary, and thyme (diffuse in moldy areas)
   - Chlorella
   - Colloidal silver (ideally the nose spray)
   - Cryotherapy
   - Follow a Bulletproof diet if possible
   - Get plenty of sleep
   - Glutathione

- Metal detox (read Anthony William's book, *Medical Medium*)
- Methyl B12 and folate (not folic acid)
- Ozone therapy
- Phosphatidylcholine (1000-2000mg of phosphatidylcholine per day with food). This can also be found in pastured-raised, soy-free egg yolks (runny). If it's not runny, you kill the nutrient you need.
- Sauna
- Selenium
- Spirulina (Vital Proteins brand)
- Up your vitamin C, E, and D3 intake
- Zinc (Bulletproof or Garden of Life brands)

To Reduce Your Exposure to Mold:
Air out new furniture if you have to buy toxic
Clean water bottles and thermoses routinely
Don't eat conventional produce and foods listed below — *period*
Handle leaks right away and make sure bathrooms are caulked well
Make and consume mold-free coffee
No air fresheners
No shoes in the home
Replace sponges regularly
Throw moldy items away — *think about papers that got wet you may have saved*
Use a great air filter — *mentioned earlier*
Use Homebiotic in your kitchen and bathroom
Wash new clothing right away before wearing and ideally buy non-toxic clothing

Avoid These Mold-Prone Foods:
Aged meats
All alcohol — *wine and beer are the worst. Organic, sulfate-free wine might be okay.*
All types of grains — *white rice is okay*

Bread
Brazil nuts
Certain cheese
Chili and other spices — *high risk, but good for you, so quality matters*
Citric acid
Coffee and chocolate — *unless mold-tested*
Corn, beans, oats, peanuts, cottonseed
Dried fruit of all types
Pistachios — *high mold risk, but very good for you if they're clean*
Pork — *unless pasture-raised*
Pre-ground black pepper — *almost always moldy*

SILENT ENEMIES AROUND US: HEAVY METALS

With dental and orthodontic work, you can ask for heavy metal- and nickel-free devices, and you should one hundred percent avoid a root canal at all costs. If you have any metal fillings, you should find a dentist in your area who does removals. You want to think twice before getting any kind of injection or implant and ensure any medical device is heavy metal-, plastic-, and chemical-free. Microblading and Botox also fall into this category of heavy metals and toxins.

Another culprit containing heavy-metals is tattoo ink. Studies show that the polycyclic aromatic hydrocarbons (PAH) have been found stored in the lymph nodes of tattooed people causing their nodes to actually turn black. Unfortunately, metals like mercury, iron, arsenic, lead, and cadmium are what give tattoo ink its color and permanency factor. Carbon Black (a form of PAH) is a soot-like product and a known pollutant, and often the main ingredient in black ink. The good news is if you're dead set on getting a tattoo, you can request vegetable-based inks (you will need to special order or request them ahead of time). If you already have tattoos, your options are to remove, or detox and up your wellness protocols.

Let's talk about the dangers of dental implants, IUDs, breast implants, and metal rods—yes, even the copper IUD can cause copper toxicity or excess copper in the body. Excess copper can create symptoms such as fatigue, nausea, depression, irritability, cravings, mood swings, and brain fog, among many others.

The most common IUD is the Mirena, and guess who it's made by? Bayer. Shocker, huh? You can find the extensive list of side effects online, like migraines, physical pain, not feeling like yourself, anxiety, and MONO-like symptoms. You can also read thousands of "Mirena poisoning" stories online. There are several class-action lawsuits against the company regarding this toxic device. If you have one, get it out as soon as possible!

> *"Estrogen dominance can be due to poor liver or gut health. Hormonal birth control can cause issues for both of these organs, which is why breaking up with birth control can be so difficult."*
> — *Dr. Jolene Brighten*

There is also a huge movement called *explanting*. Women are having toxic implants removed because they are full of chemicals, including metals, and many have been known to create mold. Yes, even saline, the "safer" ones, cause mold. The valves on these specific implants allow a backwash-like feature that can leak, allowing mold to live and grow in the implants for years. This should be taken seriously on many levels. Studies are even showing the connection with implants and cancer.

Silicone implant illness is also a thing. These breast implants are bags made of over forty harmful chemicals and can leak gel bleed into your body. It's amazing to hear the stories and see pictures of the swelling in women's faces go down, or how they look different with implants in and when they get them out; their eyes are clearer, face is less inflamed, and they feel a million times better. As stated with the Mirena, the same goes for the implants—explant them!

> *"Right now, the way I define beauty is individuality and wisdom, which I think creates a certain inner confidence. And not confidence in a way that's only on the surface, but a deep-down knowing of yourself or settling into who you are."*
> — *Alicia Keys*

While we are on the subject of breasts, I must interject this as it's plaguing our country and young minds, especially in the month of October. What exactly is the pink ribbon movement accomplishing? Are they just selling pink? Where is the education on prevention and root causes? I don't see them pointing out the connection of metals, BPA, and fragrance to breast cancer, yet they have pink ribbon perfume and lotions. *Red flag!*

How many lives have they saved? I'm all for honoring, remembering, and raising funds for a good cause, but this one just wreaks with corruption. This has been called "pinkwashing" among many informed. What does this mean exactly? They claim to care about breast cancer, but it seems they care more about pink ribbons.

The Susan G. Komen for the Cure nonprofit not only promotes a carcinogenic perfume, but they also partnered with a few companies (i.e., KFC, Yoplait, and Coke) that have products known to cause cancer and other health issues. What the actual Frank? Do you think these partnerships are actually contributing to a "cure" (newsflash: we have a cure), or are they just creating more customers for the cancer industry?

Also, how is it ethical for Susan Komen to receive donations from these well-known chemical corporations? Conflict of interest much? Komen is also pushing mammograms like they are totally safe. The reality is that mammograms only save one life in two thousand, while they harm eight to ten women through false alarms, misdiagnosed cancers, and unnecessary surgery, radiation, drugs, stress, and anxiety!

Susan is also suspected to be connected to Pharma companies and mammogram machine companies. Why isn't Susan putting money toward education, organic food programs, funding for functional medicine, alternative treatments, nutritional coaching, and immune system 101? Oh, that's right. Because that will not make her money. Shocker. *Pink flag on the play, Susan!*

Do not let anyone bully or force you to get a mammogram, keep your Mirena in, get a root canal, or keep your toxic implants. This doesn't just apply to breast cancer, but many others. False diagnoses are a real thing.

While your jaw is on the floor, how about these stats? Founder and CEO of Susan G. Komen for the Cure, Nancy Brinker, brought home a $560,896 salary in 2013. And in 2012, Komen's President was paid $606,461. Reports show this nonprofit is making $200 million per year. If you have supported, ran, donated, or even had a pink trash can, I feel your pain right now. I am sorry to shatter all your pink things. Let's take all that energy, pink, and money and give it to those actually doing good, like Children's Health Defense, EWG, and Institute of Health & Healing (pick any of the resources, programs, or doctors in the back of this book, or go order ten copies of this and pass them out). Let's host informational classes, share truths, take ownership, and say *no* to team pink ribbons.

As much as our decisions have got us to where we are in our health, the knowledge in this book, the resources, and your upgraded choices can help reverse the damage, heal, and restore. I also understand we have lived in a culture led by Pamela Anderson and the Kardashians. We have "Insta-models" and "Insta-fitness pros" (aka soft porn accounts). We have been told by every magazine cover what beauty is, but the reality is they have been lying to us all along. Photoshop, plastic surgery, and unrealistic expectations and pressures have caused so much pain within women. We see airbrushed faces and think we can't leave the house without makeup. They push the latest beauty product,

Botox, and diet that promises us "this" and "that," but leaves us so empty inside. Real beauty radiates from the inside, from intelligence, from peace, from joy, from being your authentic self, and loving yourself.

> *"I did then what I knew how to do.*
> *Now that I know better, I do better."*
> — *Maya Angelou*

SILENT ENEMIES AROUND US: EMFs

Now we are going to talk about the silent enemies of EMFs and LEDs. It's like we have created our very own *Healing Through Wisdom* language—don't worry, you can refer to the glossary in the back of the book for detailed definitions. The only giants we don't defeat are the ones we don't identify, so I commend you for sticking it out so we can slay these giants together.

Fluorescent and blue light waves are known to disrupt sleep. Do you feel relaxed when you walk into a super LED blue light building? Nope. The opposite. Yes, even those LED street lights are causing health issues. Not only are they bad for your sleep and health, but LED lights are bad for your eyes. Dr. Mercola says, "Since LEDs have virtually no infrared and have an excess of blue light, reactive oxygen species (ROS) are generated." This explains why LEDs are so harmful to your eyes and overall health. As with all we are talking about, there is an upgraded solution. You can swap out LEDs for incandescent bulbs or low-voltage incandescent halogen lights.

The reason I'm talking about lights and EMFs together is for the simple fact that certain light bulbs actually emit EMFs. LED lighting may be one of the most critical, non-native EMF radiation exposures you're exposed to daily. You know if the American Medical Association is declaring they are not good for you then it's pretty bad. When you are using these kinds of lights and exposed to them daily (think of people sitting under commercial artificial fluorescent lights all day), it can create issues such as weight issues, poor sleep quality, decreased energy, and lack of mental clarity or focus.

LED lights, along with EMFs, are affecting our biological makeup, hormones, eyes, and mitochondrial health. The lights in our homes, schools, and workplaces are not the only issue. Have you noticed those new LED street lights? They give off a horrible glare, affect wildlife, and disrupt melatonin production. Some cities, including our very own Davis, California, had their LED street bulbs removed and replaced. *Umm,* Vacaville (my hometown), expect some emails! Okay, deep breath, we need a non-LED, non-EMF, non-toxic pure air moment of silence for all of this. Are you good? Are you back with me?

If you're like me, you want to march into every FDA meeting, write letters, protest, and throw away every toxic product in your home. I feel you. That was me in 2002 post attending a Melaleuca party. Friends, it matters. All of it. I know it's a lot. We are in this together, peacefully and powerfully.

This subject is so deep and so complex I really need you to head to the back of the book to do more research. There are many summits online and in person (Bulletproof Conference and Global Summit) that cover this topic. I am going to do my best to break it down, not to overwhelm you, and to give you what you need to know and do about EMFs.

Let's start with what produces EMFs—which affects many aspects of your health, all day long. Correction: twenty-four-seven. But please note, we don't even know the rest, as we have not lived in a fully twenty-four-seven electronic age long enough to see the damage, especially on young brains.

<u>Sources of EMFs:</u>
Bluetooth devices — *baby monitors and speakers*
Cars with Bluetooth

Cell phones
Cell towers
Computers
Dirty electricity inside of walls
House alarms
Laptops
LED lights
Microwaves
MRI machines
Radars
Routers
Smart meters
TV screens
Ultrasound machines
WiFi boxes — *including your neighbor's WiFi*
X-ray machines — *especially the new ones at airports*

<u>Ways EMFs Damage Health:</u>
Affect brain function
Cause cancer and other diseases
Cause nutrient deficiencies
Damage DNA
Deplete immune system
Disrupt sleep and hormone balance
Headaches and brain fog
Heart issues — *see studies done by Martin Pall, Ph.D.*
Inflammation and digestive issues
Lower sperm or egg count — *especially when keeping phones in pockets and laptops on laps*
Stored radiation in the body
Trigger formation of cancerous tumors — *from constant lower radiation of wearable tech, such as Apple Watches*
Trouble focusing

"There's an old saying that when you put a frog in a pot of boiling water, it will react and immediately try to escape. However, if you put that frog in cool water and very gradually heat it up, the frog will 'be stuck in the comfort of its surroundings,' and stay complacent until it is too hot, and too late. This serves as a brilliant metaphor for our own human behavior and our ignorance to the rollout of technology and sciences happening in our modern age."
— *Upgrades*

A study done by Franz Adlkofer found the bio-effects of a phone over twenty-four hours were equivalent to sixteen-hundred x-rays. What the kale? Brain scans show that holding your phone up to your ear affects the neocortex and it looks like you have been microwaving or x-raying your brain. Even the American Academy of Pediatrics says cell phones are not toys because they emit microwave radiation. World Health Organization now classifies phone radiation as "possibly carcinogenic to humans," and is in the same category as lead, engine exhaust, and chloroform.

Children absorb radiation ten times as much as adults. Here we are calling it a smartphone, yet it is killing our brain cells. Thirty minutes of having your phone on or close to your head (twelve inches or less) per day increases your risk of tumors by 40 percent, and it takes four hours for your brain activity to return to normal after a two-minute phone call. Have you noticed how you feel after you take your phone away from your ear? The California Department of Public Health has warned about keeping electronic devices away from our bodies.

Dave Asprey is one of my favorite health gurus, and he is the Bulletproof and bio-hacking guy. Before he was reducing EMFs to the level he is now, he used to keep his phone in his right pocket. He says his femur has 10 percent less bone density, and he connects it to the EMFs. Crazy, right?

> *"How much more radiation penetrates our bodies today compared to ten years ago? A quintillion times more—that is a one with eighteen zeros!"*
> — Olle Johansson

<u>Symptoms of Children in High-Tech Classrooms:</u>
Anxiety
Chest pain or pressure
Difficulty concentrating
Dizziness
Fatigue
Feeling faint
Racing heart or irregular heartbeat
Weakness

It shouldn't come as a surprise when students are sitting under LED lights, have zero plants or EMF combats, and everything is running on WiFi and Bluetooth. Not to mention what is being served in the cafeteria doesn't help them with focus or health.

<u>How to Combat the Effects of EMFs:</u>
Airplane mode — *on any device not in use or any that is on your body*
Detox practices
Eat spices that support your cells — *ginger, turmeric, cinnamon*
Get tested for hypersensitivity to EMFs — *I have a hypersensitivity and need to make even more changes to decrease the risk on my own health*
Hardwire your office versus Bluetooth or WiFi
Have an expert come to your home or office to evaluate and set up protections

Keep devices in a Faraday or similar bag
Meditation and sauna
Never live near towers — *attend city meetings to deny install of new towers*
Remove smart meters — *call your gas and electric company*
Replace your microwave with a steam convection — *or use your oven and stove*
SafeSleeve or DefenderShield for all devices
Salt lamps
Shut off WiFi boxes during sleep hours
Try earthing or grounding

> *"In order for some of us to wake up,*
> *we need a wakeup call."*
> — *Dr. Joe Dispenza*

Again, here we are with vital and shocking information, and we have solutions. I do think it's crazy we are seeing cell towers popping up at schools (because let's face it, schools need money), but these towers are emitting loads of EMFs!

If you think having 5G towers on school campuses is a no big deal, consider what's currently happening with an elementary school in Ripon, California. At the time of this writing, four students have been diagnosed with cancer since the tower was placed on the school's grounds. Parents at this elementary school are demanding they remove the tower for the safety of their children, but the school cannot find a way out of their twenty-five-year contract with Sprint.

There is hope, though. The people of Danville, California fought to have their city officials deny Verizon's plan of putting a 5G tower in their town. The people were heard, and Danville rejected Verizon's tumor-tower. We should be taking a stand for this in our cities and schools. Our voices matter!

These 5G towers are a whole new level of health threat. Rumor has it, these towers are also called a "directed energy weapon." Say what? SourceWatch has even listed cell towers as a weapon of war. These towers are going up without testing this technology. We do know they produce a very high frequency, which is a huge red flag. I see a connection here to the systems. It's essential we are fully woke (what will happen to every person reading this book), and we leave no stone unturned in this journey.

Many doctors and wellness advocates have written full books covering just one of the many things listed in this section. I mention this, as I need you to realize we are just scratching the surface of these things. For many people who are already non-toxic, but still struggle in their health, I'm sure they can find the connection here. Please use caution when you want to cling to one thing like *It has to be the EMFs,* or *It has to be MTHFR,* or *It's the GMOs* and then ignore other practices or possible connections. It's important to explore, test, and try.

It's also essential we start somewhere and take steps toward healing every day. For example, you might want to focus all your attention on one enemy like EMFs and think that's good enough. I'm sorry, friend, that isn't going to heal your gut or your liver. You can change all your light bulbs, but you still need to fix those negative thoughts. You can detox from heavy metals, but if you don't eat clean, you're sabotaging that process. You can use organic, non-toxic personal care products, but if you're eating GMOs, you are missing the whole point.

I think you understand wholeness is mind, body, spirit, and even home. When I work with people in my store, and they have a long list of issues or health struggles, I help them get started by asking them what the one thing is they want to heal or see relief from most (i.e., skin, digestion, immunity, hormones, stress), and start there. You also can do the same—do things bit by bit, or room by room.

If you need to take a break to process all of this information, I encourage you to do so, as we have identified a lot of threats to our lives, homes, health, and families. Wellness warriors are rising like no other, and you are not alone. We declare war on deception, propaganda, dogma, corruption, and anything that threatens our peace, homes, health, and communities.

> *"The further a society drifts from the truth,*
> *the more it will hate those who speak it."*
> — *George Orwell*

SILENT ENEMIES AROUND US: GENE MUTATIONS

The last silent enemy is a gene mutation. I want to talk about the MTHFR mutation. MTHFR stands for methylenetetrahydrofolate reductase, which my kids and I have. In the simplest terms, it means your body can't process or convert folate, folic acid, and even amino acid into useable forms. If you have this mutation, you should *not* be taking folic acid. We are all told to take folic acid when pregnant to prevent birth defects. However, we actually need folate and not a *synthetic* form of it. Folic acid will actually block the folate receptors and not allow in folate. Not okay. This is why we are big on real, nutrient-dense supplements in pregnancy, not just over-the-counter generic synthetics.

MTHFR produces an enzyme, one I can't pronounce, to be honest, which is why it's important those with this mutation are taking methyl folate and methyl B12 (our family uses the Bulletproof brand). If you have a gene mutation or a double gene mutation, your body doesn't absorb or process key things like they should. There are variations to the mutation that I am not an expert in, but it's worth mentioning. It is also important to know this information for parents who are preparing to vaccinate their children. The decrease in the ability to detox could cause severe problems if the child cannot detox heavy metals used in dirty vaccines. Aluminum and mercury (thimerosal) do not belong in our babies. There are plenty of studies on that, and we covered a lot of how vaccines are a threat to divine health.

To test for MTHFR and other genes, you can use www.ancestry.com. Maximized Genetics or private insurance are great options, too. I will say, you are risking with testing, as you're providing your information and everything doesn't always come out one hundred percent, but testing is easy, and you can purchase the test online. You spit into a container, send it back, and wait a few weeks. Once they email your results, you will then need to download the raw data. You can take your raw data and upload it to one of the numerous sites out there to get your final results. It may sound like several hoops to jump through, but once you have your results, you have invaluable information. It's also crucial to update your providers and note your chart.

A couple of great genetic interpretation sites are:
- Dr. Ben Lynch's *StrateGene*. He gives a ton of valuable information based on your genetic data.
- LiveWello
- Some companies can test to see what genetic SNPs you may have and alert you to flagged medications for your specific mutation. For example, I have a friend who did the test through Millennium Health before a major surgery and found out Plavix could be life-threatening due to her having a homozygous MTHFR mutation. It's in her medical chart, and her doctors are aware. This is life-saving information! The more we know, the better off we will be.

<u>**Symptoms of MTHFR:**</u>
Acute leukemia
Anxiety
Bipolar disorder
Cardiovascular and thromboembolic diseases — *specifically blood clots, stroke, embolism, and heart attacks*
Chronic pain and fatigue

Colon cancer

Depression

Migraines

Nerve pain

Pregnancies with neural tube defects — *spina bifida and an-encephaly*

Recurrent miscarriages in women of child-bearing age

Schizophrenia

Healing inflammation and helping with folate and methylation, removing viruses, and pushing toxins through your body (remember, having MTHFR makes it difficult to detox or push things through, and "bad bugs" like to hang in the liver) is so vital to overall health. We can see a reversing of gene mutations when we heal, detox, push the bad out, and replace it with the good. Here are just a few ways, but this is not exact and please go back to the disclaimer: *I am not a doctor.*

MTHFR Supports:

Cat's Claw — *Whole World Botanicals*

CBD — *CW and TCH-free*

Frankincense oil — *doTERRA*

Lower fat diet — *I usually never suggest this, but for this specific gene I do*

Lysine (lowers viral loads) — *Bulletproof brand*

Methyl B12 — *Bulletproof brand*

Methyl folate — *Bulletproof brand*

More fruits, vegetables, some nuts, lots of sweet potatoes, and smoothies

Oregano oil (in capsules) — *doTERRA, Ancient Nutrition, Garden of Life, or Gaia*

Vitamin C — *Garden of Life*

Zinc — *Bulletproof brand*

Now again "bad genes" are not connected to everything, but

it's an important key. So many of the health issues mentioned above are still not understood at a deep level. I am concerned people want to pick just one silent enemy and think taking some methyl supplements will fix it all. Please know it will help, but it's not going to change everything. Dirty or bad genes are just another clue or piece to your healing puzzle, not the whole puzzle. It is also a possibility that your methyl conversion piece is connected to your liver health. Again, I am not an expert, and this whole gene topic and epigenetics is somewhat new, and there are many things still unknown.

I encourage you to look at all the gene things as a flag, sign, or piece to your journey, not the whole piece. To be clear, someone with a gene mutation—along with most humans—will benefit from a high protein and very clean diet (real organic foods, free from sugar, gluten, grains, and conventional dairy), as well as taking care of their intestinal tract, liver, and colon.

I don't believe in anyone identifying with "I have *(specific disease or illness)*" or even speaking out "I am *(negative statement)*" because conscious language is a huge part of life and a key to wholeness as well. I highly recommend reading *Conscious Language: The Logos of Now*, by Robert Tennyson Stevens, around this topic. Words have weight and power. Words create worlds. We should never identify ourselves by titles or labels anyways—be it health, jobs, or things we do. We are human beings, not human doings. Let's not be victims of our circumstances, but wise victors that change trajectories. We will be talking in detail about this in the *Mindfulness, Meditation and Mindsets* chapter. It's so important.

BIG PHARMA, BIG PROBLEMS

"Food is medicine. Pick up your prescription in the kitchen."

Now, there is a time and a place for medication, but we have an epidemic of the overuse of antibiotics, vaccinations, and prescription medications that are doing more harm than good. The other main concern is the lack of accountability, integrity, and liability from these industries. These three things alone are contributing to our suicide rates, depression rates, cancer, mental disorders, food allergies, and so much more. Your gut is your second brain, and if it's not healthy, you are not healthy.

I realize this is the part where I am labeled a conspiracy gal, and that's fine. Bless it. I also realize I am taking a risk in sharing my story, but I know that even if it helps just one person, it's worth it. Please read with compassion, and an open mind and heart. I've shared a little bit about my dad. He had significant damage done from being on prescriptions from the time he was five-years-old. He doesn't mind me sharing that he has a long list of allergies and digestive issues, along with bipolar disorder, and that is only scratching the surface.

My journey into this arena started when Gabe was vaccine-injured as a newborn. It opened me up to an entire world of corruption and a system that was doing more harm than good. (You can refer back to *From Lucky Charms to Lemon Water*.) I am not an expert in this arena, but I learned enough to make specific changes once I realized a lot of the ingredients in vaccines. There is also some moral conflict for me, as you can find aborted fetal tissue in many vaccines. *Shocking, yes. Disturbing, very.*

I also subscribe to the belief system that God gave us an immune system. He gave us the right foods in the right season. He gave us herbs, He gave us things to get well and stay well, and I need to put my trust in that more than a pill or a vaccine. Especially when that vaccine is full of things that don't mix well with allergies, gene mutations, or suppressed immune systems. Knowing all of this also meant that over the years, I had to be diligent in seeking out extra immune system supports. We don't wear shoes in the house. We sanitize with essential oils, not alcohol-based sanitizers. We take natural immune supports on top of our daily regimen, precautions, and lifestyle. We drink lots of Wellness Tea (see recipe on page 255), immunity shots (apple cider vinegar), and apply and diffuse essential oils. Even when doing a delayed vaccine schedule, there can be repercussions if the vaccines aren't metal- and allergen-free. I experienced the effects of a delayed schedule before I knew about the allergies, learning disabilities, deficiencies, gene mutations, and immunocompromisation.

I realize this is a very personal decision for people—what you eat, what you consume, what type of medical route you're going to go. I completely respect that you may have different beliefs, different ideas, different values, and a different upbringing. We both get to choose, and it doesn't have to be a debate, a right or wrong, or a friendship breaker either. *No judgment either way. Only love.*

From my heart, every word I say in this book is to inspire, inform, and empower. Nobody spends this amount of time researching, serving, living, speaking, and writing if they don't truly care. I have sat by and watched devastating things happen to people, even with their children, and sadly, it takes a crisis for them to get to the place to begin researching and making better decisions. As I described in an earlier chapter, I was in that place in 2002 when my son was hospitalized and on oxygen, while they were telling me he might not make it, and they didn't know what was wrong with him. I never want someone to be in that terrifying, vulnerable, and heartbreaking situation when it can be avoided, knowing what we know today.

Another layer to this is that I am pro-life. Again, you may believe and choose differently. We can still be friends and have honor and respect for each other. We are never going to one hundred percent agree with anyone in our life, including our parents, spouse, kids, or coworkers. There are so many levels of beliefs from faith to politics, from money to parenting, and from the economy to health, and that is okay.

As we talked about in the previous chapter, the corruption in the healthcare system is out of control. There's no denying the tie between the government, Big Pharma, abortion, and vaccines. Below is an article from Natural News. When I read this, it hit me in the gut and I thought, *"Is this America? Is this really happening?"* We can even be pro-vaccine and see that censorship, fear, and lies are unacceptable and scary to our human rights.

[A recent article] reports that Facebook announced it would block all content on Facebook that questions the official dogma on vaccines, which falsely insists that vaccines have never harmed anyone (a hilarious lie), that vaccines contain only safe ingredients (a blatant deception) and that vaccines always work on everyone (another laughable lie).

Facebook is achieving this by labeling vaccine awareness information "misinformation" or "hoaxes." At the top of the list is the assertion that vaccines are linked to autism—something that even the CDC's own top whistleblower scientist reveals to be true, yet the vaccine industry claims it's all a hoax (in order to cover up the crimes of medical violence against children that are being committed by the vaccine pushers). Also, Pinterest is blocking search results about vaccines.

The National Health Federation reports that there is a nationwide move afoot to eliminate exemptions to mandatory vaccines and to even coerce all adults into submitting to mandatory vaccinations—all in the name of "health." And that move is based solely on junk science and contrived news.

Vaccines are highly profitable for the drug companies. Merck itself makes $4.6 million a day on its dangerous and unsafe HPV vaccine. That alone should speak volumes to us about what is really behind this push to vaccinate everyone. It's not about health, it is entirely about greed.

There is zero science or facts to back mandatory vaccines for adults or for anyone. If this move to inject us all with toxic substances weren't so serious a design upon our health, it would be laughable. There is also no constitutional authority for Congress to even think about mandating vaccines. Any member of Congress who tries to mandate vaccines is breaking his or her solemn oath of office and should be expelled from office. Unfortunately, all too many legislators are willing to sell their souls for Big Pharma money.

This is some scary stuff, and it's a time in history that could swing either way. We can sit back, be quiet, and bury our heads in the sand, or we can say American rights, medical freedom, integrity, honesty, do no harm, and choices matter to me for my family and my future. Some may choose to vaccinate, and some may choose based on health screening to do it differently. Whichever your route and whatever you decide is your right. Ultimately, it's not about vaccines, but about censorship, bullying, corruption, and freedom. What's next?

You might have heard about certain conservative pages being taken down and things happening to whistleblowers and alternative health practitioners. If you don't think this is real, I have firsthand experience: it happened to me. My business page and personal page were banned from all promoting and advertising with Facebook as of May 2018. Why? We were flagged for "fake news" and "alternative health." I fought it and sent letters and years of content, showing we inspire and encourage people. They sent me a final notice saying there will not be any further discussion. We have not been able to promote any of our events, products, education, information, this book, our health summit, or even encourage people due to this. Yes, this is real.

Aside from allergies, religious beliefs, the number of vaccines in a short time given at once, the warnings inside the vaccine pamphlet, history of vaccine reactions in the family, being immunocompromised, potential developmental delays, autism, and reactions ranging from the flu, eczema, respiratory issues, and gene mutations are a main concern for many parents. Even those with non-toxic homes and mothers who are breastfeeding and doing "all the right things" might find some concerns with the current schedule.

As you can imagine, all of this drove me to dive deep into my family history based on reactions, disease, and allergies and get more testing done. My main concern was that my kids have a gene mutation, along with allergies and sensitivities, so it is risky and damaging for them to get multiple cocktail vaccines. It suppresses their immune systems and causes a variety of issues, like speech delay, mobility delay, strep throat, pinkeye, ear issues, and eczema. I exclusively breastfed them as infants, which I believe helped prevent further damage.

I think a great question to help us break down the controversy on vaccines is: Would you put all of those ingredients in a cup and serve it to an infant, a two-year-old, or even yourself? Most people would refuse. The answer is *no you would not.* So then why are we injecting poison into our bodies and expecting it not to affect or impact us negatively? I feel that my family were some of the lucky ones because I was able to reverse some of the damage done with detox protocol, prayer, education, and a change of diet. Yet, we are *still* impacted and dealing with the residual effects. My blood work shows I still have heavy metals in my system—the repercussions are no joke, friends!

If you have vaccinated or were vaccinated yourself, I don't want you to feel like it's too late, the damage is done, or it doesn't matter. It matters greatly. Maybe this is the first time you have heard about vaccine injury, concerns, or facts. I know it's a lot to swallow. Thank you for staying with me.

"I am not anti-vaccine. I am pro-child, pro-family,
pro-community. I am pro-science. I am pro-research.
I am pro-health, pro-wellbeing, pro-safety.
I am pro-government transparency.
I am pro-pharmaceutical company accountability.
I am pro-honesty. I am pro-critical thinking."
— March Against Monsanto

Let's talk about specific toxins in vaccines. Vaccines are not as safe as you may have been led to believe. I do not intend to discuss the validity of vaccines in this section. I would refer you to the National Vaccine Information Center (NVIC) and www.vactruth. com for a full discussion of this critical issue. However, I encourage you to fully educate yourself before deciding which vaccines and how many vaccines to give to your child. Regardless of your vaccine knowledge, choice, or trust, it is important to know the risks, ingredients, and how your body can be affected based on your individual health. It's also important to find a provider who will discuss this with you, offer further testing, and know your health history, all while supporting your process and decision.

Below are some of the common vaccine ingredients posted on the Centers for Disease Control and Prevention website that may shock you. Even for those that choose to vaccinate—which we all should get to choose what goes on or in our bodies—it's important to know what the ingredients are. In my world, the real "debate" isn't whether you should vaccinate or not; it's about freedom, education, accountability, choice, and safety.

Common Vaccine Ingredients:
Aluminum — *highly associated with Alzheimer's disease*
Ammonium sulfate
Antibiotics — *neomycin and streptomycin*
Calf serum protein
Cells from pig and horse blood

Chicken embryo cells
Egg protein extracts
Formaldehyde — *also used to preserve dead things*
Glyphosate
GMO yeast
Human cells from aborted fetal tissue
Mercury (thimerosal) — *especially in flu vaccines*
Monkey kidney cells
Monosodium glutamate (MSG)
Soy protein extracts

That list is concerning and *gross*, and that is only a snapshot. You can find the full ingredient list in the back. Why on earth would we put these things into our bodies, cells, and blood-streams, especially in the bodies of those allergic to many of the items listed above? If a kid has a peanut allergy, they are protected and wouldn't be forced to eat a peanut, yet why would we force vaccines that have allergens, ethical, and moral concerns in them?

The metals are very concerning as well. When I worked for Kaiser, I had to get vaccines. I asked for a single dose without metals and was told, "Of course!" That year, I got very sick and had many issues that I didn't link to the vaccines until later. Sadly, vaccine cocktails are standard. When we were kids, we got two to five "clean" vaccines. Now we have sixty-three doses and multiple cocktails. Even if you request a single dose, metal-free, or name-your-allergen-free, they are not happy or accommodating, in my experience. This is where reformation is needed.

If you're vegan, I'm sure you're freaking out seeing animal cells. We are talking about toxins known to damage the human body and the human brain. Also, think about this: if you have the cells and DNA of another human (from aborted fetal tissue) running through your blood, that might impact you in one way or another.

At this point, the main topic of concern when it comes to vaccines is that there is a lot of censorship and bullying of those who speak the truth, share their story, and ask questions. What really matters is that we each know our health history, allergies, and the ingredients. Regardless if you vaccinate or not, it is your choice. Forcing vaccines on people leans borderline communism. Sound extreme? What's extreme is removing books and documentaries on health from streaming and store platforms. Having the government tell you what you should inject into your body seems a bit insane, doesn't it? I don't think we would force Muslims to eat non-kosher, nor would we give peanuts to those with peanut allergies. You can totally be pro-vaccine and pro-right to choose.

We sit in a time in history when corruption is running rampant, misinformation is spreading, propaganda is all over, and people follow fear more than their inner wisdom. It should not be too much to ask of our system to ensure genetic and health testing before getting certain vaccines. The CDC site clearly states a whole list of "people who should not receive this vaccine." This is why we have allergy tests, medical professionals, patient rights, modern systems, and information. It's available to us so we can better our health and do what's best for each individual.

This is a very complex topic and time, but please don't accept everything you hear, read, or are told in a doctor's office. It is okay to ask questions, it is okay to do research, it is okay to change providers, it is okay to stand for medical freedom, and it is okay to talk to other moms. Above all *moms know*; let's believe them.

Whether you're a "pro-vaxer," "anti-vaxer," (enough with the labels already, for the love) or a well-informed, educated, and conscious consumer, these are things we must be aware of, expose, and change. Fighting against each other and defending our personal belief isn't going to change this system. Remember that letters, votes, phone calls, emails, texts, and respectful conversations are needed. Vaccines are not just a medical debate, but a moral, religious, and personal issue every human has a right to research and decide for themselves. If you suspect you or your family have been a victim of vaccine damage, please see all the resources I have provided for you in the back. *Remember, our bodies, our beliefs, and the things available to us are powerful and effective.*

WISDOM > FEAR

I get asked a lot how to handle knowing all this information and how to not live in fear or unhealthy emotions. To that, I refer to the power of my faith, practices, support, wisdom, and the power of choice. I can make decisions every day in my home, community, business, and family that are helping turn the tide. You might not have a company or the same kind of platform, but we all have a sphere, and most of us have social media. You are empowered.

I do need to *beg* of you to not be a crazy-conspiracy-organic-warrior that drives people away from the truth. Not everybody is ready. You can share in a loving, compelling, gracious way that allows people (ideally those searching or curious) to make their own choices.

Even when you share in the most simple, gracious, empowering, you-get-to-choose, and I-care-about-you kind of way, some people will get defensive, angry, petty, or flat out say they don't care. I have had people with cancer or significant health issues say, "I don't care. I'm not doing any of that, even if it works." That is where we know mindset, self-hate, unhealed wounds, a broken brain, and pain come into play. Their response has everything to do with them and nothing to do with you.

> *"Knowledge is power, but knowledge about yourself is self-empowerment."*
> — *Dr. Joe Dispenza*

I imagine as people are reading through this book, lights are going off and answers to prayers are happening through the words on these pages. All of it might be for you, some of it might be for you, or just one little key might be all you need. The goal is to bring light, awareness, and wisdom to some uncommon or unknown silent enemies that are preventing total health and wellness.

Maybe you already know these things or have been through some of them, and this may be something you're called to share and lead others to discover. Let us never hold back the keys to health for someone else out of fear, ego, or busyness. Someone's health might depend on your insight or experience. Do not hold back. We are at war, my friends, and we will not stop until we see a massive shift in the health of our nation on all levels. These enemies are taking lives, and affecting the quality of our families, farms, marriages, children, communities, and churches.

I hope this section serves as a guide that lasts centuries long after I'm gone. I hope you take photos of these pages, send them to friends, and reference them as you make purchases. It might need to be broken down into sections or revisited as you make slow changes. You have permission to go at the pace you need for your peace, health, and breakthrough. It's pretty shocking how simple things have now become a giant cycle of toxins, corruption, and deception. I don't believe in freaking out, living in fear, anger, or suspicion as that isn't healthy for you at all. As with anything, there is hope, resources, knowledge, and people who can help. We the people can overcome evil with good and divine wisdom.

"To beat things, we must understand things."

CHAPTER SIX

ADDICTED, BROKE, TIRED, FAT, SICK, AND STRESSED

BEYOND SICK AND STRESSED

"You can't be great if you don't feel great.
Make exceptional health your number one priority."
— *Robin Sharma*

Addicted, broke, tired, fat, sick, and stressed is about the majority of America right now. This isn't a declaration or judgment, just observation and facts. I might also add in distracted, dumbed down, numb, and delusional while I'm here.

Just find a bench in a shopping center and observe people walking by and let me know how many healthy versus unhealthy people you see (and that is purely based on appearances). We know one in five people are suffering from chronic illness, one in six are medicated, two-thirds of adults and three percent of children are obese, and nine million Americans are using sleeping pills.

To drive my point home about our prescription use, 5 percent of America accounts for the world's population, but we are using 80 percent of the world's drugs. This isn't even touching technology, alcohol, pornography, food addiction, tobacco, and illegal drugs. Addiction, sickness, brokenness, stress, and anxiety are running rampant in the wealthiest nation of the world. How can this be? This is the reality of the culture we live in. But why are we accepting this considering all we have available to us?

My heart's passion is for every person to live well, love well, and be well. We do not have to remain stuck or sick, but it is going to take making different choices, being intentional, and putting in hard work. The lines at fast food restaurants are steadily filled. The coupons sent out are for processed foods. People are not only addicted to devices and drugs, but also to food. Conventional food was made to create an addiction and keep you hungry. We emotionally and mindlessly eat, at the wrong times and for the wrong reasons. Our relationship with food is broken, but it can be healed.

"You can form new habits, you can heal, you can change."

Right now, if you look around at the number of people with healthy families, healthy bodies, healthy minds, healthy identities, and healthy emotions, you will note their life lines up with that. They are in tune with choices and overall wellness. Of course, there are many exceptions; I know I am painting with a pretty broad brush.

Every one of us is affected by these things, either personally or by those around us. We are not getting the best versions of people. Even if you're not addicted, stressed, broke, overweight, tired, or sick in some way (first off, you are an anomaly, and I'm thankful to say I'm with you thanks to the principles in this book), there are still the elements of heart conditions, the past, our heartaches, mindsets, and relationships.

People are not at their highest peak performance. They are

not reaching the potential of their gifts, talents, or overall wholeness, and it's not just them who are suffering. It's their cities, their communities, and their neighborhoods who are missing out as well. When we are not whole, we are not as useful, impactful, or personally fulfilled.

Hear me, I one hundred percent believe and know God uses broken people. He uses stories, messes, and mistakes. He uses our pain and turns it into purpose. Many people are doing incredible things despite sickness, disabilities, challenges, and pain. I am not taking away from any of that or their personal victories. I'm asking you to not just think about your own wholeness, but about what we want for our nation, our cities, our schools, our communities, our earth, our future, our families, and our future generations.

ADDICTED

"Not long ago, medical doctors endorsed, advertised for, and prescribed cigarettes to their patients. We look back at those ads and say, 'What were they thinking?' Research is now proving the epidemic rise in teen anxiety, depression, and suicide is linked to smartphone and social media use. Our kids have been guinea pigs in a tech experiment gone horribly wrong. We are facing a national public health crisis, and it's time to fix it."
— *Collin Kartchner*

Studies are just now showing suicide, anxiety, and depression are connected to social media and, specifically, smartphone usage. Imagine what will come out in the next few decades on this as we are still in the "we-don't-know" phase of twenty-four-sev-

147

en technology. I don't know if we should be shocked, as we were never made to have crisis, celebration, fear, and comparison—to name a few—all before our eyes within six seconds. What took people years to discover is now found in mere seconds because it's at our fingertips. We are being led by celebrities, sponsored brands, and influencers.

I know many are thinking, "Hey, this isn't crack, dope, heroin, crank, or speed so chill out." Actually, technology addiction is the new cigarette. Though those addictions and drugs are still very real and taking lives, the focus here is going to be on our current crisis.

Dopamine is a chemical (working as a neurotransmitter) that is produced in our brain every time we complete a task. It's supposed to keep us focused on achieving a goal or a vision. Not only is this affecting our focus, our health, and our relationships, it also greatly affects our brains.

Let's not act like this isn't the cycle: check a text message and get one happy chemical; check an email, get another happy chemical; check Twitter, another; check Instagram, another; and the vortex continues. These "happy chemicals" are shots of dopamine acquired through a cheated system. Getting a dopamine shot before the smartphone era required a lot more effort. Just as a shot of alcohol or gambling releases dopamine, the issue is that you want more and don't accomplish anything.

We have age restrictions on smoking, drinking, and gambling, but we have no age restrictions on social media and cell phones. As Simon Sinek blatantly says, "[It] is the equivalent of opening up the liquor cabinet and saying to our teenagers, 'Hey by the way, if this adolescence thing gets you down, help yourself!' "

The early studies are clear about those who are on social media more have a higher rate of depression, yet no one is doing anything about it. Over the last five years, teens have been asked if they prefer to hang with friends, text friends, FaceTime friends, or Snapchat friends, and every year, the face-to-face connection votes are going down. This is alarming.

I am very passionate about this topic as it pertains to health, as we need to control what we consume and some of the things we consume are media, music, and social media. I am one of those weirdos who thinks kids should not have smartphones until they are sixteen or eighteen. Yes, this is definitely a point of tension in our home; the balance and struggle are real. In our family, we have some simple boundaries with technology, and we are working on getting better. I'd be lying if I said we are not addicted.

"Sugar and screens are the drugs of today."

<u>Core Reasons Tech Affects Our Health:</u>
- Addiction, especially at a young age, is connected to several mental and emotional addictions.
- All the blue light and EMFs affect our hormones and melatonin.
- Best hours and days will be spent behind a screen instead of in meaningful work, relationships, and life.
- Internal struggles with identity, confidence, comparison, confusion, and FOMO.
- Lack of human connection, which is essential to health.
- Lack of communication, conflict resolution skills, empathy, validation, and encouragement.
- Not learning to cope.
- Performance and creativity are at an all-time low.
- Phones are mini slot machines in our pocket begging us to see "what we won" by the hour, robbing us of creativity, peace, contentment, and joy.
- Struggle to focus, sleep, and deal.
- Studies show a lower IQ in children and teens who use tech daily.
- The "highlight-reel" syndrome.
- These devices and apps teach us to be less than human.

- We allow social media to have too much power in our decisions and day.
- We were not meant to have this much noise all the time.

Ways to Reduce Phone Addiction and Distractions:

- Delete social media apps or move them to other pages so they aren't easy to access. (I know this is hard if you have a business.)
- Do not allow your children to have tech daily or social media until fifteen or sixteen. Honestly, I think it's best to have as little as possible. For teenagers, allow them to have one platform, discuss how it's used, check it, and allow only on weekends, not daily.
- Get a Light Phone or a "dumb" phone, and use on weekends and when traveling.
- Go a step beyond and put devices in airplane mode when they're not in use.
- Have unplugged days and take the phones from your kids. (Yeah, you can do that.)
- Leave phones out of bedrooms.
- Look into the *Digital Minimalism* lifestyle by Cal Newport.
- No phones at the dinner table.
- No phones during the first hour of waking up.
- Remove email from your phone if you have another device you can use.
- Turn off all notifications.
- Use the phone as a tool, not a trap.
- Use the screen time setting and set limits. Use apps like Screen Time or Moment, and features like Smart Family to monitor and restrict.
- Wait as long as possible to get your teens and kids phones. Pay them if you have to. I would say fifteen or sixteen might be the right age. Offer a Palm, Light Phone, or "dumb" phone instead.

> **"Addiction to distraction is the death**
> **of your creative production."**
> — Robin Sharma

I think most of us "know," and our insides are saying something isn't right about all of these screens, but the addiction keeps us trapped in the cycle and down the vortex day after day. This can be changed. I think we will look back and think, *"How on earth did we ever think this was okay?"* just as we will with much of the corruption we are living in these days.

If you implement one of the above each week and slowly wean down your screen time, you will start winning in life a lot more. I know it's hard, and especially with the kids and teenagers, but once you read the stories from *#SavetheKids*, you will never look back.

BROKE

Another downside of our addiction to phones is the cost and the entitlement to a new and better one every year. That's a great way to set ourselves up for a lifestyle of "bigger and better" in all things. Culture tells us if it isn't new, it isn't valuable. If it isn't the latest, it isn't the greatest.

Culture is a liar. I have had the same house for twelve years and the same car for thirteen years, and I love them more today than a decade ago. I admit, I have kept my old, broken phones as an act of rebellion against the system. We do not get our teens new phones, and they might not understand now, but they will later.

Do you know what the number one cause of stress in America is? *Finances.* Debt, specifically. Stress disrupts your neuroendocrine and immune systems which affect many parts of your health. We can't ignore America's number one cause of stress if we truly want to be well. Many people say finances are a barrier to getting healthy. For example, buying healthy food, going to the chiropractor, getting supplements, and getting blood work done. I understand this is a real struggle.

If we are going to combat stress in our lives, we must look at how we manage money. Without going into an entire Dave Ramsey course (which I suggest you take), I'm going to share a few insights with you.

> *"We buy things we don't need with money we don't have to impress people we don't like."*
> — *Dave Ramsey*

If you can't afford it, don't buy it. Manage your money, and it won't manage you. Living beyond our means is a major issue in this country. We "think" we "need" a better car, bigger house, more extravagant vacations, and another pair of shoes, but that's not true. We need food, water, shelter, and clothing.

Now I'm not saying to be broke and not enjoy nice things. I'm saying debt isn't the way. For me, it's a conviction as the Word says in Romans 13:8 (TPT), "Don't owe anything to anyone, except your outstanding debt to continually love one another, for the one who learns to love has fulfilled every requirement of the law." Proverbs 22:7 (TPT) says, "If you borrow money with interest, you'll end up serving the interest of your creditors for the rich rule over the poor."

I am a huge believer that wealth is greater than riches. Having an abundance mindset is a must, and we should be blessed to be a blessing. Living paycheck to paycheck, having stacks of credit cards, car payments, and overdue bills is not setting yourself up for success. It is better to have little and have peace than to have a ton of stuff with no peace.

So often you hear businesses say they are doing millions in sales and you think, *"Wow that's amazing!"* yet they owe more money than they made. That isn't real success. You will see someone with a new house, new car, and taking vacations (again, these are good things when managed well) saying they make a certain amount of money, but they own none of it, and their debt is more than they are worth.

It takes major self-discipline not to blow your check on a new outfit when you have bills to pay, especially when you're young. I get it. A lot of people were not raised or taught how to manage money, how to budget, or even the value of a dollar. Thank goodness there are so many supports in place that can help you live and get debt-free.

Basics to Live a Financially Abundant Life:
- Be mindful of your purchases and the "why" behind them. Many people use money as a sense of control as it makes us feel powerful and releases dopamine.
- Don't take on student loans if possible.
- Downsize and take a minimalist approach.
- Get out of debt if you're in debt, and even plan to pay your mortgage down in fifteen years instead of thirty.
- Have a budget and know where your money is going. Use apps like YNAB, Mint, or EveryDollar.
- Live generously. We have tithed for twenty years, even when we were broke, sharing a car, and low on groceries. Blessings are not just money, but health, working appliances, running cars, and peace.
- Make things last by taking care of them and don't buy new unless it's necessary.
- Plan ahead for emergencies, vacations, and holidays.
- When money comes in, it should go to tithe/giving, bills, emergency, savings, debt, then spending. It's important to teach our kids these principles, too.

Happiness doesn't come from wealth, but wealth can come from happiness. Angry, grumpy, tired, sick, and negative people are not usually wealth builders. A sure way to decrease and stop stress is to begin to manage your resources. Start with a budget, then plan to pay off debt and go from there. If you want to live an excellent, abundant life, you must be willing to make excellent decisions in every area. I'm cheering you on as you take one step toward freedom, health, success, and true abundance in every area.

TIRED

> *"Sleep is the golden chain that binds*
> *our health and our bodies together."*
> — *Thomas Dekker*

How many people are saying *I can't* to themselves and others due to a few things:
1. They can't afford it (the trip, the concert, the holistic coach, or the course).
2. They are too tired.
3. They are down with a headache and can't show up.
4. They have stress, anxiety, or depression guiding their decisions.

This is now just culture's norm. It stops here. Something mainstream we hear often is, *"I'm sick and tired of being sick and tired."* We can agree that too many people around us are laid up with colds, back pain, migraines, and coughs. They are exhausted and lacking light, energy, and clarity. Thankfully, a lot of the answers to these things lie within the pages of this book from changing your environment, mindsets, heartsets, habits, and lifestyle.

Based on research and what everyone in the "health" world agrees on, *sleep* is essential and the one major thing that can pack the most punch to bettering or worsening the status of your health. Sleep is a big topic as over fifty million Americans are struggling with their sleep, and nine million are using sleeping pills "to help." The worst part is placebo studies have shown the sleeping pills aren't working, and the side effects are horrific.

Understanding the benefits of sleep and how actually getting *quality* sleep is essential. Being in bed and sleeping is not the same thing. No matter what, everybody sleeps; it's the one thing happening across the world that we all have in common, besides breathing. Sleep is essential and vital.

> **"You're not healthy unless your sleep is healthy.**
> **Enough sleep is more vital than exercise."**

When you are sick or stressed, the top suggestion is to *get more sleep*. Yet no one is taking this golden advice seriously or hacking their sleep. Instead, they are ruining it by doing all the wrong things to try and sleep well. So many of the issues we talk about in this book would be significantly improved if sleep quality was improved.

It's a great step to take individual responsibility for our sleep, but we can take it one step further by hoping to see change in schools (later start times for teens), government (take away the time change, as it's proven to do more harm than good), and businesses and corporations (having the right lighting and supportive environments). We will continue to have a clear "sleep crisis" on our hands as a nation if steps are not taken in these directions.

We all know we are hardly any good to ourselves and to others when we are exhausted. It costs corporations productivity, families deeper connection and peace, our teenagers extra stress, and a decline in health for many around us. We can change it with action and execution of some pretty simple things—some of which are free or a one-time cost—to greatly improve sleep quality.

"Exhaustion makes wimps out of us all."

Basics of Sleep Cycles:

Light: This makes up about 50 percent of our sleep, and it begins a sleep cycle.

REM: REM is regulated by circadian rhythms (your body's internal clock and rhythm). This cycle of sleep is so important as it's the phase we dream. Dreams are a part of our creative process, and they are a way we get "self-therapy." Sadly, but not shockingly, sleep aids and pills block REM sleep. We are a medicated sleep society from sleeping pills to screens, and alcohol to melatonin. This stage is all about memory consolidation, learning, and dreaming. It can be anywhere from 5-50 percent of your sleep.

DEEP: The most restorative session of the night, and a must for full recovery and detoxing. It enables muscle growth and repair. It makes up about 0-35 percent of your sleep.

For those of us incorporating exercise into our lives—as it is a must for *optimal* health—we may be tempted to push ourselves in workouts when we didn't get optimal sleep. We are better off taking it easy or adjusting our workout that day for lasting wellness.

You should sleep based on your personal circadian rhythm. Studies show if you take anyone to camp for three days, including those with insomnia, when they go to bed around sundown and get up at dawn, all insomnia was gone, and their clock was regulated. Most believe sleeping from 10:00 PM to 6:00 AM is the average best. Again, this is very personal. Ideally, my body loves to sleep from 9:30 PM to 4:45 AM, and around seven hours and twenty minutes is my sweet spot. You need to test, try, and apply different things to find your best sleep rhythm. As a general rule, it's best to get six to eight hours of sleep and ensure you're getting the right amount of all three phases.

"Prioritizing good sleep is a great act of self-love."

Better Sleep Habits and Hacks:

- Additional sleep supports: Sleep Mode, Uncorked's Dream supplement, Garden of Life's sleep drops, Trace Minerals magnesium spray, Vital Proteins collagen sleep shot.
- Don't take a nap past 3:00 PM.
- Get thirty minutes of natural sunlight per day or try red light therapy, such as Joovv Go.
- Get your circadian rhythm aligned.
- Go to bed early or in alignment with your personal circadian rhythm.
- If you drink caffeine, don't have any past 2:00 PM.
- If you use an alarm, ensure it wakes you up with soft music or something calm.
- Keep a journal by your bed.
- Keep exercise to morning hours or at least three hours before sleep.
- Make sure room temperature is right (63 to 68 degrees) and try non-toxic temperature regulating sheets, like Ettitude.
- Make sure there are no WiFi boxes or smart meters near your room, in your room, or outside the wall of your room. Keep your room tech-free if possible, and your devices in airplane mode.
- Set your mind and intentions on when and how you will sleep and wake up.
- Stick to a sleep schedule as much as possible with the goal of six to eight hours of sleep.
- Stop eating three to four hours before bed. Practice eating a large breakfast, medium lunch, and light dinner. Try fasting

from 7:00 PM to 7:00 AM, or the time frame that works for you.

- Use white nose, essential oils, CBD, magnesium, and black-out shades to improve sleep.
- Wear an Ōura ring and understand how to use the data.
- Wear blue light blocking glasses.

The great news about sleep is you get a guaranteed chance to improve and adjust it every night. You can start this today!

> **"Early to bed and early to rise
> makes a man happy, healthy, and wise."**
> — *Benjamin Franklin*

FAT

Exercise is likely the most widely accepted and known keys to health. You see, before our modern world and in other current cultures, life was exercise. For example, hunting, climbing, walking miles each day for resources, running from danger, and carrying supplies for miles. Clearly, we are not going miles for water, carrying animals over our backs, and climbing up hills with heavy equipment. The reality is most of us spend half of our day in a car or at a desk, which we know is harming our health.

Thankfully, we are now hearing about this everywhere, and people are getting standing desks, taking walking lunches, installing windows (indoor light and air is also harmful for extended periods), and allowing exercise balls at desks. The goal isn't just exercise, it's also movement. This is a great start for sure. Again, your health is really 80 percent what you consume (food, products, thoughts) and 20 percent fitness. I'm not taking away from exercise, but it's important to note you can work out seven days a week and still be unhealthy.

I think many people are overwhelmed by how, when, and

where to exercise. When things seem complicated, we tend to avoid them. We also think we need to kill ourselves in the gym to see results, which just isn't true. We have all tried things from CrossFit, spin, sports, machines, and programs, and didn't stick it out long enough to make it a habit. Friends, sixty-six days is the golden number for instilling a lifestyle change.

For some people, they have not found what works for them, what they love, or how to overcome the mental blocks that keep them from breaking through in this vital area. There are countless resources on exercise and the benefits, so I leave that to the fitness experts and gurus. I will briefly touch on some great health benefits and resources for you.

First are two programs to help you understand which fitness style works for you: DNAFit and Diet Fitness Pro. We need to be sure also to have lots of non-exercise movements in our day, as well as get in at least ten thousand steps per day for optimal health. Exercise and movement vary greatly, so it's important to understand your body, your current health, and goals.

We know exercise helps with sleep, stress, digestion, and hormones. It also boosts your mood, extends your life, lowers your risk for many diseases, promotes neurogenesis (growth of new brain cells), reduces anxiety and depression, lowers your cortisol (the fear hormone), increases BDNF, increases serotonin (the chemical that regulates happiness), increases energy, builds confidence, boosts levels of dopamine, increases anandamide levels (neurotransmitter and endocannabinoid produced in your brain that temporarily blocks feelings of pain and depression), and boosts your immune system.

Now, there are many more benefits, but that is a general foundation to the amazing benefits you will get from regular exercise. As much as there are many forms of exercise, I strongly believe we should have a variety of exercise in our routine instead of doing the same thing every day. It's proven to improve your goals and health, as well as prevent injury.

<u>Commonly Asked Workout Questions:</u>

How long should I exercise and what are some workouts? I recommend working out twenty to ninety minutes per day, depending on the workout and your overall personal wellness. You can do a quick twenty-minute routine at home right when you jump out of bed at 5:00 AM (remember, the 5 AM Club is key), and do jacks, planks, push-ups, sit-ups, or yoga. There are also a ton of free videos on apps and Apple TV (such as Chalene Johnson or BBG). You don' t need to have a gym to work out. Hop on a bike, or go for a run; just move.

When should I exercise? I suggest and prefer mornings or early afternoon. Late workouts affect your sleep quality.

What is your workout regimen? This varies week to week, but here is an example: I listen to at least two podcasts during my workouts. I drink 20oz of lemon water before I go, another 30oz while working out, then 20oz after. As I mentioned, I fast 7:00 PM to 7:00 AM most days, so I don't eat before I go. Also, some days I do a twenty-minute workout at home before my reflection and learning time (part of my 5:00 AM 20/50/20 method).

Monday: 5:30 AM cardio or home HIIT (mix it up), weights (arms), squats, and planks.
6:15 AM sauna and meditate. I also get in ten thousand to thirteen thousand steps throughout the day and take my dog on a walk a few afternoons each week. I also do things with my kids like play catch, roughhouse, etc.

Tuesday: 5:30 AM cardio (bike and elliptical), weights (legs), squats, and planks.
6:15 AM sauna, and some Tuesdays I will go lighter if I'm going to a spin class at 9:15 AM.

Wednesday: 5:30 AM cardio (row, rope, incline, and sprints), abs, and barre.
6:15 AM sauna, meditate and stretch. I also go on a prayer walk from 8:00 to 9:00 AM every Wednesday with friends.

Thursday: HIIT, light cardio, arms, then sauna, meditate, stretch, or take a TRX class. At night, I play volleyball for an hour.

Friday: I don't work out every Friday, but I ensure to get in a walk, sauna time, and at least some Yin Yoga, or I take the day off, depending on what my Ōura ring data says.

Weekends: Walk dog, stretch, and a few weekends a month, I will get in thirty to sixty minutes at the gym depending on our travel and work schedule.

I personally love SPRINT (a fast HIIT spin class), barre, my own system of cardio and weights, TRX, and certain yoga classes. I was mixing in three classes a week when I did my workouts past 8:00 AM. Sadly, a lot of classes are not available at 5:30 AM. I'm also not a yogi like most would think. It's a goal of mine to get better at it, but it's not my BFF; everyone responds and engages differently.

I would suggest investing in a personal trainer or doing a challenge for at least four to six weeks before you try to go on your own. Once you no longer have a class, challenge, or trainer, you should still have a workout buddy or accountability. When working out becomes a healthy habit, you will begin to see the benefits and sometimes actually enjoy it. The key is to prepare by laying out your clothes the night before and getting up right away, before the excuses set in.

*"How you feel after a workout is never
how you feel before the workout."*

161

WISDOM DOESN'T TAKE A DAY OFF

If you've been in the health and wellness or fitness space at all, or even if you follow people in the space, you're probably familiar with the term: "cheat days." Let me start this by saying I believe in treating yourself. I do *not* believe in cheat days, as people use them as excuses to set aside their convictions, their allergies, their standards, and their hard work all in the name of a toxic meal that isn't worth it.

Now, there are those of us who believe in treating yourself, where you might eat something you wouldn't usually eat on a day-to-day basis, but it still fits within your values and standards. Mine, for example, might be when I go to Pushkin's (a local dairy- and gluten-free bakery). I would consider that a treat for me because even though it's clean, it isn't something I'm going to have every day. Another might be getting a paleo donut at my favorite coffee shop (shout-out to Journey Coffee). Again, it isn't something I'm going to do every day, but I call it a *treat*, not a *cheat*.

What blows my mind is people who say they're into health and wellness and wholeness, yet they eat McDonald's or Taco Bell or Starbucks on their cheat day and celebrate it! Many call this "balance," and I get where they are coming from, but it still doesn't line up.

I truly believe we are leading people the wrong way when we say, "Hey, let everything go on this day." That is a slippery slope, not just with food, but (in my humble opinion) with morals and values, as it pertains to other things as well. There is something to celebrating, traveling, or being on vacation, but compromising what you believe and what's good for you in the name of those other things doesn't seem legit. You know very well those things are going to inhibit all the hard work you've been putting in, and they're going to make you go back to day-one if you've done a detox or an elimination diet. They are also going to wreak havoc on your system because it's been cleaned out! When you put chemicals, toxins, and foreign things into your body once it's been cleaned out, your body is like, "What are you doing to me?" This is why when people try to go back to eating like crap after they've done Whole30, GAPS, paleo, or keto, they feel terrible.

This should be a huge signal that our body was designed to eat well and to feel well. It's dependent on us to choose well. This is why I don't believe in diets; I believe in lifestyles. It doesn't make any sense to be disciplined Monday through Saturday and then on Sunday, throw everything out the window and go through a vicious cycle of discomfort and other symptoms so you can eat some fries. Now, if we're talking about homemade, organic sweet potato fries, I'm all for it.

The other part of this isn't just about the food or what's in it. Again, it goes back to what we are supporting and what we are voting for with our dollars. I do not want to give to something that goes against everything I believe in. I also don't want to sabotage my own breakthrough and growth and feeling amazing just so I can have some In-N-Out. I promise it really isn't good after a while, and honestly, I don't feel like I'm missing out one bit.

I want to encourage us to change the mindset from cheating to *treating*. We should absolutely celebrate, reward, and enjoy the things that are delicious and designed to nourish and fuel us. I very much enjoy chocolate chip cookies (*Against All Grain* recipe), waffles (*The Whole Food Diary* recipe), ice cream (raw from Be Love Farm), and a paleo donut (from Journey Coffee). No one is missing out around here! We are choosing upgraded, elevated, Garden-versions of goodness! So friends, stop having cheat days, promoting cheat days, and throwing all your hard work out the window in the name of vacation, celebration, and attention. We can and will do better! Lasting change, next level mindsets, total healing, and wholeness belong to the dedicated and disciplined.

"Stop suffering and start stewarding."

UPGRADE YOUR CHOICES

So much of our depression and anxiety are not only connected to food, environment, toxins, gut health, and our thoughts, but to *where* we are living (past, present or future). Erwin McManus says, "When you're living in the past, you're depressed. When you live in the future, you're anxious." This is why living in the now (being present and mindful) is so important.

If you're depressed, aside from the other facts shared in this book, you are likely living in the past, and you believe the lie that your future will be like your past, which can be summed up as hopelessness. My dear friends, the keys to freedom are in your hands, in your pantry, in your mind, in your words, in your meditations, and in your daily decisions.

If you apply these tools along with the many other valuable truths weaved through this holistic encyclopedia, you can trade addicted for free, broke for blessed, tired for rested, fat for fit, sick for well, stressed for peaceful, and you will not only change your world but those around you. Let's do this.

CHAPTER SEVEN

DEAR CHRISTIANS

*"I believe that the greatest gift you can give
your family and the world is a healthy you."*
— *Joyce Meyer*

Let me talk to Christians and people of faith. Let me have a heart-to-heart with the Church (this means the whole body of believers, not one denomination or church).

You might be asking why I'm "calling out" or speaking to a specific faith group. It's because this is my faith group. It's my upbringing. It's my culture. It's my family's culture. I think this message can apply to many faiths, schools, and systems, but I want to be clear where I'm coming from. This is also where *Healing Through Wisdom* came from, in a sense. I was tired of seeing people get the same Sunday prayers but make the same Monday decisions. (Can I get a witness?)

Here's the thing, if you are not a believer, religious person, or Christian, I don't know if it will be beneficial for you to read this part, but you can if you want. I don't want it to be received or taken in the wrong way, so that's why I give this disclaimer.

Having been raised in the church and a Christian my whole life, I feel this is an essential message to my fellow believers. It could very well be the game changer we all say we've been praying and waiting for. We all know someone, even incredible pastors, songwriters, worship leaders, and authors, who have dealt with health challenges. Some of these health challenges have taken those people out, and some people have overcome them.

The three who come to my mind are Doug Addison, Beni Johnson, and Jim Goll. These are very prophetic pastors and intercessors who I respect as they went through their health challenges. I have attended their conferences and read their books, and they are the ones I know who chose the alternative health route. Through that, they became advocates of natural health and have helped many other people see that healing is not just through prayer, environment, forgiveness, and meditation, but also through taking specific action. Before I go any further and have a Charismatic freak out on me, *take a deep breath*.

I entirely believe spiritual attacks can happen in our minds, bodies, and spirits. There are plenty of Bible stories to back this up—Saul, Paul, and Job are a few. It's also happened to me. Warfare is real. So is wisdom. I would highly suggest reading *Spirit Wars*, by Kris Vallotton, if you have struggled or been under torment of any kind.

I believe that Jesus can heal. He heals today, and He healed when He was here. I do not discredit miracles or healings at all—I pray for them, I have seen them, and I am a huge believer in them. Part of the calling on my life is to be an intercessor; I love prayer, and I have seen God answer many prayers. I do not take away from any of that.

There is not only one avenue to healing, just as there is not only one avenue to hearing God, experiencing supernatural things, and getting insights and revelations. You can hear God through the Word, a dream, an impression, another person, worship, a sermon, meditation, prayer, in nature, and so many more ways. We must not limit ourselves, our faith, or the roads that may bring us into new encounters.

MY THEOLOGY ON HEALTH, SICKNESS, AND GOD

Allow me, friends, to describe some truth to you, and what my theology is on sickness and healing: God doesn't give what He doesn't have. Your sickness or disease wasn't given by God or caused by God, and it isn't your cross to bear. I believe God heals, restores, and redeems all things—cities, places, people, dreams, families, emotions, hearts, health, and lives. I believe He gave us all we need to be whole, well, and to run our race.

God knew what He was doing when He made fruits, vegetables, nuts, plants, and barks. I think the Native Americans lived this best, along with the pioneers. They had raw milk, healed cuts and wounds with lavender and aloe, and everything was organic. Sure, there was some ignorance there, too, like contaminated drinking water and sanitation, but you get the point.

> *"There is power in partnering with what God created and intended to heal and nourish."*

How can we be set apart when our divorce rates and health rates are the same as what's happening in the world? What makes us different if the numbers come up the same? I realize that is a blanket statement, and of course, there are many things the Church and believers are doing brilliantly. I am a product of the Church, so to say, and I am proud of the incredible work being done.

I believe and know and have seen God heal (be that emotional, mental, spiritual, or physical—it all has value and weight). What I am hoping to get everyone to consider is that although He is in the business of hope, health, and healing, He is also in the business of wisdom and stewardship. My Bible says our body is a temple, and sadly, I don't believe many of us are following that principle. Do you know that way back, people lived for hundreds of years? Have you ever thought about how or why? I have. I came to the conclusion that it was because everything was organic and the environment wasn't toxic. Yes, they still had flawed and broken humanity, but the earth, food, air, soil, and the "system" wasn't what it is today. I truly wonder if we were completely free of chemicals in our homes, bodies, hearts, minds, and nature how long we could actually live. Yes, He heals, but He also reveals!

TRINITY OF HEALTH

> *"Don't let your temple betray your destiny*
> *—take care of your physical body."*
> — DeVon Franklin

Many people believe in the principle of sowing and reaping, or as culture would call it—karma. People like to talk about this principle when it comes to everything else besides our health. I'm no math expert, but I can just add up years of consuming food (which is really more chemicals than food), on top of all of the toxic products we use in our home and personal care routine on a daily basis, and eventually, we are going to reap from those decisions. We accept the fact that if someone smokes for a certain amount of years they will get lung cancer. Simple, right? Why do we not then believe that what we put in our bodies, minds, homes, and spirits have the same effect?

You could also say something is going to eventually manifest within our body, mind, or spirit due to what we have been feeding it and how we have stewarded it. If we do not have physical health, if we do not have spiritual health, if we do not have mental health, how do we plan to be impactful? How do we plan to build strong families and communities? How do we plan to be what one of my favorite proverbs says? "Wise people are builders—they build families, businesses, communities. And through intelligence and insight their enterprises are established and endure" (Proverbs 24:3, TPT).

It's a bit difficult to innovate, have insight, build, and create if you are not living or feeling your best. So many people focus on what their calling or purpose is, and I think that is noble and important. I believe we each have a destiny and an assignment that is unique and powerful to only us. I wonder, though, what would happen if we took the same amount of energy we put into our purpose and we put it into our health, wellbeing, and our wholeness instead. I think many people would be much more clear on their purpose and calling because they would be operating at a higher level, mentally clear, productive, powerful, and peaceful. I have found people who feel great make great decisions and do great things.

I have also seen people who may call themselves "spiritual" or "enlightened" depend solely on certain practices—be that crystals, sage, or meditation (which as you'll learn, I'm so down with meditation)—as their sole source of getting peace or healing, but ignore the trinity of health. They may practice the spiritual things, yet they're still going through the drive-thru on Tuesday and putting toxic products on their bodies, and they think the spiritual practices are the only things that matter.

This also goes for fitness gurus. They're doing a great job pounding the protein, amino acids, getting to the gym, and their bodies may look incredible, but are they checking the ingredients in their shakes and fitness supplements? Are they taking care of their spirit and mind as well? As much as working out is great for your mental health, brain, body, and spirit, it's really tying all those things together that leads to optimal divine health.

I can say with confidence that Jesus and His disciples were not breaking toxic white bread and pesticide fruit from a land full of chemicals. I can also confidently say that God knew what He was doing when He crafted and created the Garden and gave Adam and Eve stewardship over it. Friends, this might be breaking news, but there were no GMOs in the Garden. Coca-Cola, Clorox, and McDonald's were not growing on trees.

I believe in the Makers Diet—be that more plant-based or grass-fed, sustainable, animal product-based, or a mix, as long as it's within the realm of original design and creation. When there is a real, original design (the purest version), you will always find a counterfeit, contaminated, copycat version. Just look at identity, marriage, farming, and health.

I don't know about you, but I want real in my life. I want to eat real food, I want to have real friends, and I want to serve a real God. I believe God designed organic food for our nourishment, our strength, and our development. He knew what was best, but our nature as humans is to get involved (which sometimes is a great thing—we should be co-creators) and turn into co-controllers where we compromise what was originally designed for our benefit.

> **"Your fork is the most powerful tool
> to transform your health and change the world."**
> — *Dr. Mark Hyman*

There are many churches with a heart for excellence; they want to have the best lights, the best sound, the best coffee shop, and the best lobby displays, and I am in full support of that. Let people create excellence! My concern comes when we completely neglect excellence in our health when it comes to food and taking care of our mind, body, and spirit. There is a lot of teaching in churches on the Word, values, and commandments—absolutely necessary things—but we also need to teach people about how to care for and steward their bodies, minds, and spirits.

Often, we commission our community and our church congregation to change cities, the school system, and the music industry (which is all great—let's add our unique creativity and anointing and all of that to those arenas), but why do we not first focus on being a person of value? A person of help. A person not numbed out on medications. A person with a ton of energy. A person who sleeps well. A person who is secure, confident, bold, and brave.

I have seen the inside, or "soul health," of a person neglected and overworked at the expense of a gift, creativity, or service. If we really want to maximize people's potential, we must increase the attention we are giving to their health. Let's set them up to thrive. When we put candy, chips, and donuts in front of people, we are making it easy for them to fail. Yes, people have free will, but we can set them up to choose well. We may want to consider what we are serving in children's church. In this day, when one in ten people have some type of allergy, I believe it can create a conflict for parents and their children when they have to tell them "no" to the candy other kids are eating.

I say all this, but I completely understand and have been guilty of this, myself. When my sons have hosted small group, I have bought the pizza they requested because, quite frankly, they didn't care enough to have anything else. I also recognize cost is a factor when you are feeding hundreds or thousands of people. The cheap route is to grill the hot dogs and get the pizza. I understand that.

There is a way around this because *community* is about bringing our resources together. I know we are all busy and we just want things taken care of, but what if as a church at the next youth gathering, instead of having pizza, we called on a few different people to add something to the table? Serving in this way brings some people life. Remember, we want to spend, eat, and share intentionally and mindfully. We can also plan things outside of meal time and focus more on conversation.

I know what you're thinking because I'm also thinking it:

This just isn't practical. I realize we have some considerable barriers to cross before we're in that place. It is hard for me to understand why we have donut walls at women's and men's conferences, and then we don't understand why people are not fully engaged, or why they have to leave because they have a headache, or why they come down with a sinus infection the next week. No, that one donut isn't the culprit, but it certainly isn't adding to health and wellness. The majority of people are in the state of mind where it's normal to them, and they would see a donut wall as amazing—I respect that. However, the number of people who are turning down the donut wall is growing. We also must consider having something else to offer to those who have allergies, or those with high convictions around what they put in their bodies. Now, if the donut wall is paleo, save me one.

> **"If you want to feel great, be great,
> and make an impact, you have to
> make great choices."**

I often have believers (even people who work within a church) come to me with their physical complaints, post on social media that they're sick again and picking up their antibiotics, and complain their kids are sick, but they refuse to attend an annual health conference, listen to a podcast, read an article, or do some research. Some even go as far mocking and making fun of people who are into organic and wellness. People have poked fun at my lifestyle, my calling, and my convictions. I understand I choose to live differently, and I'm okay with that. What some don't understand or respect is the majority of people adopting this lifestyle have battled or suffered from diseases or allergies.

The Church does a great job talking about the power of our thoughts and how we need to renew our minds. That is biblical! We also love the scripture that says to focus and meditate on all things that are good and holy. Those things matter and are essential, but it's harder for some people when their gut is not healthy (there is such thing as the gut-brain connection), they have damage to their neural pathways, or they don't realize or believe in neurogenesis. So many believers are left feeling discouraged and frustrated because they are trying to implement these powerful biblical principles *mentally* when really there is a strong connection between our health and minds. The healthier our bodies are, the stronger our minds will become, and vice versa. The stronger your mind is, the stronger your heart will become.

I don't think we should do the work for other people, but I do believe we need to give them every tool to enable them to do the best job possible. If you were to ask someone to make a cake and only provide them with a pan and one ingredient, they're going to have a hard time. When we're asking a congregation to do X-Y-Z, but we're not giving them the X-Y-Z tools, we set them up for frustration and failure.

Let's be real though, so many people want the easy way or others to do the work for them. We can't want something for someone more than they do, or work on their problems harder than they are willing to. That is codependency. It's one thing to empower and support, but it's another to micromanage, manipulate, and control. At the end of the day, everybody gets to choose, and we, in turn, get to choose to accept people right where they are. We can't make anybody sick, and we can't make anybody healthy—that is up to them. Their daily choices determine that. However, we can diligently make sure the options we offer are ones that line up with sustainability, health, and wholeness. I believe we are called to steward our time, resources, bodies, minds, gifts, and communities well.

We see our culture is staying in so many of the same cycles, and some of it is due to the system. We create systems that support codependency, or we create systems that support a poverty mindset. It's a wonderful thing to want to help those in need and to trust the process, even when things don't line up or make sense. We are responsible for our part. I love that the Church is helping the poor, supporting widows, visiting people in hospitals, coming to people in crisis, helping make schools better, and creating amazing prison ministries—all of this is incredible, and I have so much respect, love, and honor for it! I can only hope and wonder what would happen if we began to incorporate health as a core value, and if we started to empower every one of these areas with healthy options. What would our churches look like if we gave our people the knowledge and education to help them understand their daily choices and their physical health is impacting their mental and emotional health as well?

I have this crazy thought: If you're going to buy something anyway, why not buy with purpose and intention? If you're going to eat something, why not eat things that were intended for your good? If you're going to do something, why not do it with all your heart, soul, mind, and strength? If you're going to be effective, you might want to be informed, educated, inspired, empowered, and fully woke so you can go the distance. My heart for health is for us to be empowered to make better decisions, feel better, live better, serve better, love better, and choose better. This will take looking at things we don't want to, and giving up vices and unconscious decisions. It requires awareness and intention, but the fruit of it is a strong and healthy mind, body, and spirit, which leads to healthy families, communities, and cultures. It's bigger than us.

I believe that we should walk in conviction on how we steward the earth, our home, our families, our finances, our thoughts, and our bodies. The goal is the trinity of health—mind, body, and spirit—all being healed, acknowledged, fed, awakened, nurtured, and managed well.

CHAPTER EIGHT

MINDFULNESS, MEDITATION, AND MINDSETS

"Health isn't just what you're eating, it's also about what you're thinking and saying."

I love sharing about wholeness as it pertains to our mindset, heart health, and emotional wellbeing. As mentioned before, you can eat the kale and take the probiotics, but if you don't deal with what's going on with your heart, you're not truly well.

A big part of becoming an adult is unlearning a lot of the shiz you were taught by people who didn't know what they were doing or how to be whole themselves. This is not an excuse or card to play, but a reality we must accept and learn from. Where this book takes the gold medal is that we are going way beyond food and exercise. We are going much deeper than a few good quotes and stories. These tactics, methods, applications, and wisdom will take your life to a whole new dimension if you allow them. It's time to cut out the noise, lies, sabotage, fear, excuses, and negativity, and take your life back. The future belongs to those that are willing to change it.

"If you get the inside right,
the outside will fall into place."
— *Eckhart Tolle*

MINDFULNESS: THE BRAIN AND WOO WOO

Buckle up! Later in this chapter, we will talk about the basics of meditation and contemplative prayer and how you can have a mindful meditation practice. To be really clear, mindfulness and meditation are not the same. They can be talked about like they are, and many current buzzwords can make all this seem confusing.

Mindfulness is simply being aware of the present moment, as well as what you are experiencing at the moment. It isn't woo woo or complicated. No magic wand or crystal ball required.

Another word that can get tossed around in this context is *mantra*. A mantra is a tool of the mind. It is a word or symbol used to ground and center yourself, also known as an affirmation. We should be our own biggest fan and cheer ourselves on. I love practicing "I Am" statements in my journal and out loud. I also love to get a word from the Holy Spirit every day to center on. *Decree* or *declaration* are other words you can use for mantra. Of course, everything is what you make it and the place you're coming from.

Manifest is another buzzword often used. To manifest is to make clear or evident, obvious, apparent, plain, and put beyond doubt or question. For example, manifesting your dreams or your best health is going to take time, work, and discipline. We will also talk about this a little later.

Another term that gets tossed around along with these words is the *law of attraction*. You know how when you decide to get a Jeep you start to see them all over the place? And how when you begin to learn about organic it shows up everywhere? Simply put, that is the law of attraction.

"You make room for and magnify what you focus on."

If we want to truly have better mindsets and see results from all this "brainwork," we might want to understand a bit about it first. I believe we have more power within us as co-creators than we understand. When you are praying for something (and working for it), there is a basic checklist use:

- Are you being specific, positive, and clear? *Vague prayers get vague answers.*
- Does this desire serve your highest good, benefit all involved, bring glory and honor to God and your true self? Does it align with your calling?
- Do you have three confirmations and green lights?
- Are you aligned with this, claiming it, receiving it, and also surrendered (not attached)?

Think in terms of days, numbers, people, and locations when being clear in your prayers. Specificity has power, as does surrender. I'm a huge believer in writing things out, so make sure your goals, dreams, and desires are written. I believe God loves to answer prayers and partner with us in our purpose, passions, and productivity.

Now, there are also different types of prayer, and there are plenty of books on this topic listed in the back, but for clarity sake, intercession and prayer are not the same. *Intercession* is when you are praying for others and standing in the gap for people, places, and history. I love prophetic intercession.

The last word I want to talk about here is *consciousness*. Consciousness is to be aware, awake, sensitive to, and responding. I have no idea why people get all weird about this word. There are four stages of consciousness: wakeful, sleeping, dreaming, and transcendental.

This consciousness is not to be confused with the two minds we have: conscious and subconscious. The first (conscious) consists of the thoughts we intentionally choose to think. It's 5 percent of our daily behaviors. Shocking, right? The second (subconscious) controls how we see life, react, what we think about ourselves, and what we think we can accomplish. It is programmed and conditioned on each thought, action, emotion, and experience we've had in our life. It is the part that is running you 95 percent of the time.

It's important to address two things as it is *very* possible to change the structure of your brain (neuroplasticity) and create new brain cells (neurogenesis). It's important to understand this as we are not our genes or our bodies, but we really are our thoughts, beliefs, emotions, and agreements.

John Paul Jackson was one of my favorite prophets, and he had a great teaching on this. It is important that we take ownership of our thoughts, energy, frequencies, and words as it pertains to our lives just as much as our choices. Things are not "just happening," and the quickest way to fall into a victim mindset is by asking, *"Why is this happening to me?"* versus, *"What is this teaching me?"*

Research has shown 75-98 percent of mental, physical, and behavioral illness is caused by our thoughts. There is so much more to this and DNA, and there are amazing experts with fantastic books on this subject you should check out. This is one of my favorite topics, and I believe there is much more we will discover in the future on this fascinating wisdom about the brain.

I also want to mention our prefrontal cortex, which is usually talked about when a teenager makes a poor choice, as it's not developed until age twenty-five. The prefrontal cortex allows you to observe your own thinking and allows you to choose how you will handle a situation or circumstance. This is why it's so important to be *conscious* and have a healthy brain. Did you know you can self-regulate your thoughts every six seconds, and you have about sixty thousand thoughts per day?

Let's go real woo woo and talk about the pineal gland and brainwaves. We addressed this briefly when we talked about fluoride in *Enemies of Health*. Your pineal gland is located in the center of the brain. This tiny organ regulates your daily and seasonal circadian rhythms.

We also have different brain waves (frequencies). Throughout the day in your waking state, your EEG will display all five types of brain waves at once. However, one specific brain wave will be dominant depending on the state of consciousness you are in.

Your brain has constant electricity running through it. These electrical signals work with chemicals (dopamine, serotonin, oxytocin) to influence how you experience the world. A brainwave is the pattern of electricity your brain generates, and there are a few different kinds of brainwaves:

<u>Gamma:</u> Gamma waves appear to be involved in higher brain activity, which includes perception and consciousness. While you're in this state, your brainwaves range from zero to four cycles per second.

<u>Alpha:</u> The frequency of Alpha is a mental state of deep relaxation and meditation. It is the bridge between Beta and Theta. Alpha is what allows you to daydream, visualize, and gives you a state of consciousness that is detached and relaxed. As Dave Asprey says, "Alpha waves give you a feeling of deep calm, coupled with productivity, creativity, and effortless focus." When we are in a state of physical and mental relaxation, even when we are aware of what is happening around us, Alpha frequencies are around seven to thirteen pulses per second.

<u>Beta:</u> Beta is the brainwave state where you are active and alert. These frequencies emit when we are consciously alert, or we feel

agitated, tense, or afraid, with frequencies ranging from thirteen to sixty pulses per second.

<u>Theta:</u> Theta is a state of very deep relaxation; it's also what happens during REM sleep. The brain waves are slowed down at a frequency of four to seven cycles per second. Theta waves are always creative, characterized by feelings of inspiration, and very spiritual. It is believed that this mental state allows you to act below the level of the conscious mind.

<u>Delta:</u> This is a state of unconsciousness, deep sleep, or catalepsy. Delta is the state of mind when you're in a deep sleep. In Delta, brainwaves are slowed down to a frequency that varies between zero to four cycles per second. It is also the wave that you use when the phone rings and you already know who's calling.

Scientists have discovered that certain brainwave frequencies (especially Alpha and Theta) may:
- Relieve stress and promote a lasting and substantial reduction in people prone to anxiety states.
- Facilitate a deep physical relaxation and mental clarity
- Increase verbal ability and performance IQ.
- Better synchronize the two hemispheres of the brain.
- Recall mental images, and spontaneous, imaginative, and creative thinking.
- Reduce pain, promote euphoria, and stimulate the release of endorphins.

Brainwaves matter, as they can be a huge part of your healing, effective prayer, and meditation, as well as personal growth. I listed binaural tones in *A Day in my Holistic Life*. You can get an app, a Wholetones box, or a headband to enjoy this kind of sound therapy and get "dialed in" more every day. Brainwave support isn't just for meditation, but for sleep, focus, creativity, healing, and so much more.

My final thoughts on the brain are regarding the left brain, right brain myth. Yes, we have different parts of the brain, and they have various functions. I was raised to believe that the left brain is more logic, math, and admin focused, where the right brain is more emotional intelligence and creativity. There are times we engage certain elements more than others, but that doesn't mean the other parts are inactive. They actually work simultaneously. As we know, the brain is not cement, and it can change. Effective thinking involves both sides of the brain. Dr. Caroline Leaf has even explained in depth how the mind and the brain are not the same things.

Another brain myth is that we only use 10 percent of our brain. Many people also say you have the brain you are born with, and intelligence is pre-determined—wrong. You have the brain you work for. I would highly suggest checking out Jim Kwik for more on this.

There are also supplements, meditations, and practices that can improve and heal our brains. You are not a victim of your current brain. Often times, we love to use labels and statistics like, "Oh such-and-such runs in my family," or "I am a Di or an Eight on the Enneagram," or "I'm more right-brained," to justify where we lack. I know this as I've been guilty of it, myself. The truth is that every heart, mind, brain, body, and spirit is capable of wholeness, change, and healing. Nothing is beyond restoring or changing. Knowing your triggers, your pains, your strengths, and your weaknesses will enable you to identify the root and rise above it. Instead of playing the "blame card," "victim card," "brain card," or "family-history card," why don't we play the "put-in-work card," "God card," "prayer card," "I-have-tools card," and "anything-is-possible card?" As my pastor often says, "If you don't quit, you win."

MEDITATION

"Tranquility is the new luxury of our society."
— *Robin Sharma*

Meditation is reflection, prayer, pondering, daydreaming, and deep thinking. It is centered, aligned, and focused thinking. Meditation trains your brain to focus, rewire, receive, process, be still, and heal. It also involves relaxing the body, calming the mind, going beyond wandering, thinking, looking inside, and—for those of faith—looking up. Some call meditation the eighteen-inch journey; it's going from the head to the heart.

Don't worry, it isn't sitting in perfect stillness, quiet, and having zero thoughts. Mediation has been around and practiced for a long time. Meditation is also biblical. Certain meditation practices are rooted in religions and beliefs. It's nothing to be afraid or intimidated by; just because we don't understand something doesn't give us permission to dismiss it or judge it.

We may have also been given the wrong idea or information about mediation. I understand if it's new, it might feel hard at first, but as with anything, it's something to practice, and you will get there. As with journaling and writing, something is better than nothing, and meditating for five minutes is better than not doing it at all.

Health Benefits of Meditation:
- Boosts immune system and decreases chances for other health issues
- Calms your amygdala (the part of your brain that makes you crazy)
- Helps dump toxic stress and emotions
- Helps improve and naturally treat learning disabilities, such as ADHD
- Helps recover from illness and injury faster

- Improves focus, performance, and cognition
- Improves sleep quality
- Increases neuroplasticity: you don't have the brain you want, you have the brain you've earned
- Increases positive thinking, reactions, and responses, including more empathy and compassion for yourself and others
- Increases productivity and decision making (clarity)
- Increases willpower and self-control
- Less anxiety and depression because of the stress reduction
- Promotes emotional health and gives space to bring things into your awareness, including repressed emotions and old wounds
- Reduces stress and lowers cortisol levels
- Twenty minutes of meditation is equal to one additional hour of sleep. When paired with sound therapy (binaural tones), it's double that. We know how important sleep is to optimal health and recovery.

"When thou prayest, shut thy door; that is, the door of the senses. Keep them barred and bolted against all phantasms and images. Nothing pleases God more than a mind free from all occupations and distractions. Such a mind is in a manner transformed into God, for it can think of and understand nothing, and love nothing except God. He who penetrates into himself and so transcends himself, ascends truly to God."
— *Albertus Magnus*

I am not a meditation guru, though I do meditate daily and practice at least three of the ones listed next each day. I know there are many more types and styles, these are the ones I have practiced and am familiar with. You may also combine a few during your meditation time. For example, you might start with gratitude or worship, then focus on your breath, then a scripture or word, then practice self-compassion, and maybe end with a guided meditation. Or you might flip all that and start with a guided meditation, then finish with intentions, gratitude, and a mantra. The formula is what works for you, and that might be based on the day and your emotional need. You may also find you stick to one type of meditation that works for you. My only suggestion would be for you to be open to trying some of the others I list as well. One common theme in any form of meditation is learning to bring yourself back to center. It's normal to get distracted or have your thoughts go lots of places. This is why we call it a practice. There is no failure in your personal practice, only adjustments.

Types of Meditation:
<u>Guided:</u> Using an app like Calm, Soultime (Danny Silk's are my favorite) or Headspace, you are led through meditation. You can also be led by a facilitator, like a yoga teacher or coach.

<u>Spiritual, Prayerful, Inner Healing (Contemplative Prayer):</u> A meditation time that is centered around prayer and inner healing. This is where you can work with God through pains, trauma, and more. In Christian tradition, the goal of contemplative prayer is for moral purification and a more in-depth understanding of the Bible, or a closer intimacy with God.

<u>Soaking:</u> This also falls into spiritual or Christian meditation. Some call this *waiting on God*. The focus is really to rest in God, focus on Him, yet not strive. You might turn on some worship music, leave a notebook nearby, and wait for a word, verse, direction, or vision.

<u>Scripture:</u> Taking a verse and really focusing on it, its meaning, its power, and how to apply it to your life and the world around

you. Giovanni, from the Live & Dare blog, says, "*Lectio Divina* literally means 'divine word' or 'divine reading.' It involves choosing a short passage from the scripture, memorizing it, and then repeating it silently for a few minutes. During practice, all ideas, thoughts, and images related to the passage are allowed to arise spontaneously in the mind. It is somewhat in between contemplative reading and contemplative prayer."

Gratitude and Mindful: Focusing on all the things you are thankful for and noticing all senses at work and around you.

Focused or Breathwork: Making the focus of your breath a picture or object to help increase the amount of time you can focus without distractions. Relaxation meditation is great as well, and involves body scans and relaxing different muscle groups at a time.

Movement: Walking meditation, gardening, hiking, etc.

Prophecy, Decree, or Mantra: Taking a prophetic word that God or someone gave you, a quote, or an affirmation, and saying it out loud, seeing it, and focusing on it. You can even write it down, read it several times, and pray over it.

Self-Compassion: Not exactly a meditation, but can be seen or practiced as a form of meditation or done during your meditation time and visualization. It can be executed in even one to three minutes while driving or doing dishes. For deeper healing, it's best done when you are more focused. It does speed up the process of rewiring the brain, which is essential to heal the mind. I share in detail about self-compassion in the next chapter. For now, note that self-compassion on your own or with God is a powerful tool for deeper healing, preventative health, and staying in a powerful mindset over a pity mindset. Self-compassion is releasing empathy, validation, kindness, and assurance to yourself, your circumstance, pain, situation, or struggle. The main goal of self-compassion is to change your chatterbox (your daily self-talk).

VISUALIZATION

***"It has been said that the body
will embody what the mind is visualizing."***

We use visualization as a tool to prepare our physical, mental, and emotional state for high performance, increased immune function, or better sleep. Meditation can calm your nervous system, where visualization can reprogram it.

Most meditation is focused on being restful, where visualization can be more active, though they can both be practiced together. Visualization is also known as *guided imagery*, and many spiritual people use the word *vision, prophetic,* or even *picture.*

It is so powerful, some even practice it and call it *daydreaming* instead. The reason it works is that we use the same part of the brain to picture the action as we do to perform the action. When the focus of meditation is an image, the meditation becomes visualization. Visualization is sometimes called *mental imagery* or *mental rehearsal,* too.

Some even call this type of meditation *setting intentions.* Intentions are a goal, an aim, or something intended. Intentions are set daily, though you may or may not be aware of them. Meditation time is a great time to set intentions, as we talked about earlier in this chapter.

The famous quote by Alan Lakein, "Failing to plan is planning to fail," comes to play here. If you don't set intentions, get really clear, picture the outcome, responses, and breakthroughs, then you're not playing at a hundred percent. As an athlete and someone who loves sports, I have read and listened to countless studies on the greats, and it's not only their work ethic, skill, talent, and coaching, but so much of it is their belief. Many of them practice visualization.

One study took a group of basketball players and had them practice shooting an extra hour. They took a second group and had them meditate and visualize for twenty minutes and practice for twenty minutes. I bet you can guess the result. Yes, the ones who practiced less but added visualization made more shots.

Russian scientists have proven visualization's effectiveness by conducting a study that compared the training schedules of four groups of Olympic athletes. Each group used a different combination of physical and mental training:

Group one:	100% physical training
Group two:	75% physical training
	25% mental training
Group three:	50% physical training
	50% mental training
Group four:	25% physical training
	75% mental training

The scientists found that the fourth group performed the best during the Olympics. This is incredible, inspiring, and should make everyone want to visualize their best day, life, marriage, family, job, talk, church, and health.

In sports, you will often hear that what happens at practice determines the win, and what happens "in there" determines what happens "out there." I know we love a good name drop for reference—LeBron James, Michael Phelps, Novak Djokovic, and Derek Jeter have all shared many times about their meditation and visualization practices. What athlete wouldn't want to boost their confidence, composure, clarity, and have an extra advantage?

We should never underestimate the hours of practice, discipline, work, and training, though. When my son played baseball, a common term his coaches used was "see it." I have applied this to my life, business, dreams, relationships, and situations. As a radical dreamer, I can tell you I have *seen* a lot come to pass, but there is far more to come as well.

This book was in my spirit and mind's eye before it was in your hands. To get even simpler with this, when I have my morning rituals and practices, I also visualize how my morning will go with my kids, how I will respond to their humanity (aka sass and drama), or what interactions I will have with customers and friends. I also use this for podcasting, writing, events, and when I play volleyball. (Got to get those strong serves, ya know?) My son has used this as a multi-sport athlete, and my daughter always "sets her intentions" before horseback riding. And of course, we include prayer in that, too.

Now, here is where people get tripped up. They think they should picture Lambos and millions of dollars and it should just happen. This isn't even close to what I am talking about here. I also realize life happens and people are human, even when our routines are on point, we meditate, drink Bulletproof coffee, take the supplements, say the affirmations, set the intentions, and align ourselves. Here's the deal, we can't control anyone but ourselves, and all of those things you practice do matter and enable you to handle the flat tire, rude guest, cranky kid, and bill in the mail with peace, confidence, grace, and awareness. This is a huge win, and you can remain a peaceful warrior instead of a pity party victim.

I know firsthand how powerful "seeing" is. I know that pictures don't come as easily, but it can be learned. Even now, close your eyes and picture a red balloon—see you can do it! It takes intention, awareness, guidance, and time. Remember that picturing is engaging one sense, but add in the emotions, feelings, sounds, smells, gratitude, and praise as though it has happened. The challenge is not being attached to it in an unhealthy way. It's a fine and sacred dance, but the more you dance, the better you get.

PRAYERFUL MEDITATION

"When we don't nourish ourselves with fresh,
healthy food, restful sleep, regular exercise,
a daily spiritual practice, such as meditation
or journaling, and other mind-body healing
habits, we will inevitably feel tired,
out of balance, irritable, and
sometimes even depressed."
— *Deepak Chopra*

I want to dig a bit deeper into prayerful meditation. Prayerful meditation is when we have a desire we want to happen (manifest), and we want to surround those thoughts with surrender, belief, and gratitude as if it already happened. You can picture (visualize) this desire coming to pass and generate the feelings of excitement, celebration, and the emotions connected to that. You are not just sending up words and waiting around; you are actively participating in prayer.

Remember, we are co-creators. There are even studies on people who pray and meditate, called neurotheology. It's shown that the brains of those who spend consistent time in prayer and meditation are not the same. Dr. Caroline Leaf says, "Twelve minutes a day of focused prayer over eight weeks can change the brain so much so that it will show up on a brain scan."

The other fascinating thing researchers have found about meditation is that intentional thought for thirty seconds affected laser light (frequencies). Frequencies are nothing crazy, just basic science. Sound is a frequency, your heartbeat is a frequency, we are a frequency. Positive emotions emit positive frequencies, and negative emotions emit negative frequencies. These are measured by your personal energy field. Don't run for the hills, sit tight.

As much as the food we eat (more frequencies), thoughts, daily choices, environment, and emotions are crucial, the emotions we have affect our energy and frequency. To put this plainly, high frequency is higher health, and low frequency is lower health. The power of gratitude, positivity, and love—as talked about through this book—actually enables and turns on your body's healing systems. How amazing is that?

We also know the energy we carry is *felt* in the atmosphere we are in, so we can raise the vibration (energy and frequency) of those around us by carrying gratitude, peace, love, hope, and joy. We know words, thoughts, and deeds that produce positive feelings bring you and those around you up. And it seems to be obvious that the words, thoughts, and deeds that draw out negative feelings bring you and others *down*.

Ultimately, in many ways, we are all connected. How we live our lives not only affects us but those around us. This is why I'm committed to speaking hope, life, and truth to those around me and to myself. I am also deeply committed to being a culture changer, future creator, and an innovator in the area of wholeness.

> *"When you renew your mind,*
> *you also renew your emotions."*
> — *Andrea Thompson*

MY PERSONAL PRACTICE AND EXPERIENCE

I'm a seer, so I get movies, pictures, and visions. That is me. Others have different experiences. Some are more feelers, knowers, or hearers. However, as I mentioned, anyone can learn to visualize, set intentions, or do guided imagery.

I learned an amazing meditation from Father Richard Rohr that I practice at least once a week. He says to imagine you're on a dock or beach. There are ships or boats with large sails near this dock. You then take your current problem, pain, frustration, stress, or situation and put it on the boat and watch it sail away until it's out of sight. I also like to pray a prayer of trust and surrender about that thing and visualize God taking care of it. I love to wave goodbye to my stress, problems, grace-growers, and worries. It is so freeing and powerful.

Here are a few other examples:
- A lot of people use the ocean waves coming and going as a meditation to keep them centered on a rhythm.
- You can have a quick visualization of a chalkboard with limiting beliefs, circumstances, or pain listed on it, and then visualize yourself taking an eraser and wiping it all away, replacing it all with truth and positivity.
- When taking a shower, you can imagine the water is washing off all your cares, stress, concerns, and circumstances.
- Focus in on one word or phrase (i.e., Jesus, God is able, peace, love).
- When I practice self-compassion, I also check in on all my "roles" (i.e., mom, wife, writer, business owner, speaker). Sometimes one part of me needs more attention than the other. I like to spend time acknowledging, affirming, and loving on each part of me. If something feels off in me, I often times do a quick scan to check in and can find that the mom part of me is feeling a certain way. I then handle that quickly.
- I love to practice affirmations, mantras, and decrees—so much so I listed many that I use in an entire chapter.
- I also really love walking meditation.
- Throughout the day, I make sure to check on my breath. I will also do some de-stress breathing as well. This is a basic practice I have used in my doula practice, called an *exchange breath*: Breathe in peace, strength, and healing. Exhale stress, confusion, and tension. In addition, I will do a quick body scan on my shoulders, hands, neck, and posture.
- I sometimes open and close meditation with prayer, as it is a partnership and an addition to my spiritual practices. (Me-

diation does not replace prayer at all though.)
- I love to picture a big, open box. I put every problem, every word, and every to-do list in the box before bed. Then, I watch God walk away with the box and say, "Good night! I've got this. I'll take care of it so you can go to sleep."
- The last one I want to share is meditating on prophetic words, promises, verses, and even revisiting old journals.

MINDSETS

How many of us have said, "If I would have known that then, I would have done so many things differently?" I mean, I don't think I learned how to properly communicate a need until I was twenty-five. For example, "I feel lonely and isolated, and I could use some one-on-one time together."

Now, I'm not a therapist, but I do love all things healing, and I have not just learned a lot but applied what I've learned from therapists, mentors, coaches, and my personal experiences. I have been able to use these principles to heal from rejection, irrational and negative emotions, emotional neglect, betrayal, abandonment, hardships, loss, and life.

> *"Journal to awaken your mind*
> *and transform your life."*
> — *Asad Meah*

As we come into contact with our pain, thoughts, dreams, greatness, and struggles, it's important not just to know the options, but how to apply them. Journaling (with pen and paper, not a device) is one of the most powerful and free tools with great benefits like:
- Alignment
- Brain rewiring

- Clarity
- Creativity
- Healing
- Immunity
- Positivity

> *"What happens to us is not as important*
> *as the meaning we assign to it.*
> *Journaling helps sort this out."*
> — *Michael Hyatt*

I use a very basic but effective journaling strategy every day. You can take what works for you and try some or try all, but know that writing something is better than writing nothing. When I was homeschooling my middle son, I made a pre-formatted note for him in his daily log like:

I am thankful for *(three to five blank spaces)*.
I am *(three to five blank spaces)*.
I will *(three to five blank spaces)*.

My practice is similar, but has a few more elements:
- I bullet down my dreams from the night before.
- I write down ten things I'm thankful and grateful for.
- I write three to ten "I Am" statements or affirmations.
- I write down three to five people I'm praying for.
- I write a decree for my day or situation.
- I write my top intentions and priorities that day.
- I write a scripture of the day. I also like to write a few lessons and thankfuls in my journal before bed.

You can also journal out thoughts, ideas, feelings, and much more. There is no limit or exact formula. What matters is that you make journaling a part of your everyday life, and you will see your everyday life reap the benefits of this simple yet powerful practice.

> **"Journaling is paying attention to the inside
> for the purpose of living well from the inside out."**
> — Lee Well

Here is a summary of all the mental, emotional, and spiritual health practices:

- Acceptance
- Clean system and home
- Counseling, coaching, or therapy
- Detachment
- Exercise: *you only need twenty minutes to get a good sweat, increase BDNFs, and release stress*
- Forgiveness: *self, past, others*
- Gratitude: *it's a game changer*
- Healing: *mindsets, beliefs, wounds, toxins, toxic emotions*
- Holistic lifestyle habits: *see full list in* Holistic Must-Haves and Pantry Swaps
- Journaling
- Meditation: *twenty minutes a day, two times a day*
- Perspective shift
- Purpose and passion
- Routine: *see* My Holistic Habits *on page 45, plus systems like time-blocking*
- Self-care: *see full list in* The Power of Self
- Self-compassion: *practice at least three times a day, and on the spot as things happen (hurt feelings, rejection, offense, pain, abandonment, betrayal, stress)*
- Sleep: *six to eight hours with three cycles (light, REM, deep)*
- Spiritual practices: *read the Bible, attend church, find a small group, be accountable, declare God's truth, worship, meditation, affirmations, prophetic ministry, contemplative prayer*

> *"Acknowledging your emotional state is*
> *an important tool in supporting all*
> *of your other health goals."*
> — *Dr. Mark Hyman*

Detachment doesn't mean not caring. It's taking care of yourself first and letting others take responsibility for their actions without trying to save or fix them. That sentence alone is a great setup to address co-dependency, *but* I will leave that one alone, as you can find tons of resources about that topic. Attachment is the need for ownership, and detachment is a sense of appreciation. For example, you can love and appreciate a cool piece of furniture in a store window, but not have to go in and purchase it. You can see flowers and appreciate their beauty, but not have to pick them.

Attachments also can come as perceptions or expectations. When we hold on to things so tight, they are a cause of pain. The more mindful and present you are, the more aware you will be of not just your state, but if you are moving toward attachment or detachment.

> *"Unexpressed emotions will never die."*
> — *Sigmund Freud*

The habit of suppressing emotions is a threat to our emotional health, and we must pay attention to it. In simple terms, suppressing our emotions is like saying, *"Oh whatever, I don't care!"* when something happens, hurts you, or offends you.

As powerful as positive thinking is, you cannot keep ignoring your feelings and emotions deep down inside that you think you have forgotten about or don't matter. They will always arise later, and they manifest in many ways from anger, addiction, avoidance, abuse, and beyond. The worst way they can manifest when paired with victimhood is self-hate. Your mindset and intelligence can be off the charts, but if your heart is broken and toxic, you will not step into the full greatness you're capable of.

> *"Time only heals the wounds*
> *you're willing to work on."*
> — *Rob Hill Sr.*

Ways to Heal Emotionally:

- Acceptance
- Acknowledge
- Create an emotional outlet
- Compassion
- Detachment
- Develop tools and skills to cope
- Empathy
- Express your emotions (crying, dancing, running, journaling, punching a pillow)
- Forgiveness
- Find your purpose
- Let go of the past
- Practice self-forgiveness and self-compassion
- Reach out
- Spend time on passions and hobbies
- Take your time
- Tell your story and share your journey
- See self-care list in the next chapter

> *"Not being present is a sure thing to eliminate.*
> *Being present allows you to maximize the*
> *moment and the energy of the people,*
> *place, and God's presence."*

One of the most powerful lessons you will ever learn is how to channel the negative energy from the pain you have suffered into constructive actions that improve your life and the life of others. Using the things mentioned here, like meditation, binaural tones, and journaling, are really key. It's also important to find ways to embrace and celebrate the negative; find the gold in the dirt, and the wisdom in the wound.

> *"Your life is as good as your mindset, choices, heart health, and spiritual condition."*

How to Change Negative Thinking, Limiting Beliefs, Anxiety, and Stress:

- Ask yourself if it's a possibility or certainty. *Is it one hundred percent happening?*
- Ask yourself if you're making something bigger than it is.
- Ask yourself if you're over-analyzing something.
- Eliminate toxic thinking, speaking, and words (i.e., can't, try, need, but).
- Exchange the negative for the positive, and the lie for the truth.
- Find out where your thoughts are from and whose voice they are (i.e., ego, enemy, wound, someone else).
- If it's a picture, replace the image (reject, rebuke, replace, release).
- Instead of clinging to it, let it pass, and send it back where it came from.
- Is love or fear your counselor?
- Is this fact or a false and limiting belief?
- Remind yourself what and who you have control over: *yourself.*
- What does God say about your situation?

Benefits of Counseling, Therapy, or Having a Life Coach:

- Ability to set boundaries
- Better relationships
- Greater self-confidence
- Increased assertiveness

- Less anxiety
- Regained emotional balance
- Trauma resolution

> *"Fall in love with taking care of yourself.*
> *Fall in love with the path of deep healing.*
> *Fall in love with becoming the best version of*
> *yourself but with patience, with compassion,*
> *and respect to your own journey."*
> — *Sylvester McNutt*

How to Stay Healthy in Your Mindsets:

- Allow failures and pain to become fuel as you fail well and heal fully; failures are a part of the growth process.
- Be aware of your ego and pride speaking and rising up.
- Be aware when you are in your old self versus your new and true self.
- Continue to develop your gifts, vision, and passions.
- Stay in a place of process, growth, and true identity.
- The true you knows who you really are: *positive, peaceful, productive, powerful, and present.*
- Transform every wound, pain, and lack into healing, wisdom, hope, freedom, and authority.

It is very hard to say what I feel to be the most powerful or favorite part in this book, but I do feel very strongly about the power and practices that have been shared in this chapter. I have seen these practices do miracles in my heart, life, circumstances, and health. The power within ourselves is incredible and the emotional states I've seen people grow through using these tools have been nothing less than transformative.

I get fired up talking about mindsets and effective tools for your wholeness. I truly believe what lies within these pages should be taught in schools. As you read on into the journey of self, it is only an added piece to perfectly go together with what

198

you have just discovered. Take a deep breath, relax your shoulders, and minimize your distractions as you are about to go even deeper.

Becoming the healthiest version of you takes time, you will get there. Purge the behaviors that are holding you back. Improve your strengths and develop your weaknesses. Make sure self-awareness is always present as you go through this growth phase. You can do this."

— *Sylvester McNutt*

CHAPTER NINE

THE POWER OF SELF

YOU: YOUR MOST IMPORTANT RELATIONSHIP

*"The most important relationship you have
is the one you have with yourself."*

I have found one of the most powerful parts of my wholeness journey has been getting to know, understand, heal, take care of, and transform myself along with old patterns, programming, and wounds. It's hard to change anything you're not aware of, and if you don't have the love, confidence, skill, or mindset, you may find yourself circling the same mountain. I'd love to see you dive into each of these and really discover new strengths in yourself. I'm going to overview them before we briefly unpack into some effective practices.

The Powers of Self:
Self-confidence: positive self-belief, assurance in your personal ability, power, and judgment.

Self-compassion: offering empathy, kindness, and understanding to yourself.

Self-motivation: ability to do what needs to be done.

Self-management: managing your internal and external worlds.

Self-forgiveness: extending grace and forgiving yourself for choices and behaviors.

Self-awareness: awareness of your personality, character, decisions, and actions.

Self-love: regard for your wellbeing and happiness.

Self-care: a form of care and management for quality of life.

Self-worth: a sense of your value; the basis of your thoughts, feelings, and behaviors.

Self-talk: the conversation you are having with yourself all day long.

Self-sabotage: behavior that blocks your breakthrough, healing, blessing, or goals. For example, procrastination, self-medicating, repeating cycles, and being stuck in limiting beliefs.

Self-hate: extreme dislike, judgment, shame, and guilt in yourself. Even feeling anger toward yourself. This usually leads to projection onto others, self-sabotage, and some studies show the connection between autoimmune disease and self-hate. Robin Sharma says, "Procrastination is an act of self-hate."

In this moment, think of three things you love and you are thankful for. Write them down here:

_____   _____

_____

Now, as you look at them ask, *"Why didn't I list myself?"* So often we have been conditioned to think it's arrogant, prideful, or narcissistic to care, love, and comfort ourselves. Being selfish and arrogant is entirely different than practicing the "powers of self."

You can certainly hit the gym, be in the 5 AM Club, pursue mastery, eat kale, and take supplements, but if you're harboring bitterness, self-hate (usually stemming from not living out your gifts and potential), negative self-talk, being hard on yourself, and having intense self-doubt which also leads to self-sabotage, you will find that total freedom and wholeness doesn't come easy or last.

> **"If you plan on being anything less**
> **than who you are capable of being,**
> **you will probably be unhappy**
> **all the days of your life."**
> — *Abraham Maslow*

We often worry about things outside of our control, what others are doing, or how we can fix others when the focus should start and end in a healthy way with ourselves. Victims love to blame and make excuses. As my friend, Gayle Belanger, describes, "Victims also JERD (justify, explain, rationalize, defend)." We must understand the diseases plaguing humanity are victim-itis and excuse-itis.

Yes, you probably had a bad childhood, that teacher was toxic, that partner was negative, and your boss was a tyrant. No one is diluting that. The key here is that you are responsible for you. You can control your thoughts, feelings, actions, words, emotions, and decisions, despite what others are or have done.

You have a self-critic and self-champion. Some people also call your self-critic your conditioned self, false self, or your ego, and your self-champion your true self or authentic self. People also call them your small self and highest self, or old man and new man. However you want to put it, we are daily at war with which "self" is showing up and which "self" is thinking and talking. This is why it's great to ask of your thoughts, feelings, and words, *"Which voice is that?"*

As emotional intelligence, quantum physics, and neuroscience are exploding, you can find much more information on this topic. If you're ready to walk in your purpose, be healthy in your mind, body, and spirit, and succeed in life and relationships, this is the truest foundation and place we must begin.

SELF-AWARENESS

"Know thyself."
— Inscription from the Temple of Delphi

In some circles, the "powers of self" come off ego-centered and cocky, but it's truly the opposite when you open up and dig into them, starting with self-awareness.

This is something tossed around and maybe not always understood. Some assume you either have self-awareness or you don't, which in some sense can be true. For example, a lack of self-awareness might be when you think of the person who goes on American Idol or The Voice, and they truly believe they sound great, but they don't. They could use a little self-awareness in that situation, or maybe some truth-tellers in their life. Some people may be self-aware just not easily embarrassed. This is usually true of those who are an Eight on the Enneagram, as we tend to be very self-confident by nature.

Understanding yourself is such an essential for growth, healing, and change. I don't think we should blame or identify everything with our particular love language, StrengthsFinder, DISC profile, Myers-Briggs type, or Enneagram number. I think these are incredible tools we all need not only for ourselves, but to understand others better as well.

"If you don't know who you are
or what you stand for, the world will tell you."

We often hide behind the vision of our spouse, job, parents, or other people, and we don't step into who *we* are meant to be. Supporting, partnering, and serving someone you know you're called to is holy, sacred, and amazing. I'm not taking away from that. Where it goes sideways is when we use that as a way to hide.

Many times, mothers will keep getting pregnant and have another baby because they don't know who they are or that they have value outside of being a mother. They want a baby but forget the baby will be a sixth grader one day. It's only a temporary fix and place to hide. Young people are hiding behind the degree their parents want them to have, and parents are hiding behind their kids' sports and schooling.

Some can also take their titles and labels much too far— mom, husband, boss, athlete, writer, and friend. Those are what you are doing, not who you are. We are human *beings*, not human *doings*. Your identity isn't a title or label. You are loved, loyal, passionate, compassionate, strong, beloved, treasured, sacred, kind, and generous.

Yes, we have personalities, and those are our gifts. Being creative, talented, loud, and gracious are not just accidents; our gifting lines up with our callings. Please know my heart is that these things matter and are holy, but when they are your excuse not to be you, there is a problem.

> *"If we are not conscious, we are unconscious.*
> *When we are unconscious, we lack self-awareness."*
> — *Scott Jeffrey*

Being self-aware is a practice of owning your strengths and weaknesses. Self-awareness also builds emotional intelligence (EI), which is essential for success. Another layer of self-awareness is our habits. Sometimes we form habits, and it takes others to help us realize what we are doing (i.e., interrupting others when we talk). To everyone I have interrupted, please forgive me. I'm a work in progress. Once someone points it out, we usually become more conscious and self-aware so we can then change the habit.

Self-awareness can also get wrapped up in identity, as some people are still discovering who they really are, aside from titles and labels. We don't need to be coached by culture, friends. Being your authentic self is being your most powerful self. Who you are is an essence; it is eternal, and it is vital to our history.

SELF-LOVE

> *"You must love your neighbor*
> *in the same way you love yourself."*
> — *Mark 12:31 (TPT)*

Know thyself. Love thyself. Self-love isn't selfish; it's wisdom. It's not the same as arrogance or pride. Too often we wrap ourselves up in false humility and put our own mind, body, and spirit on the back burner, and we wonder why we're burnt out. We need to be our own biggest fan, comfort, cheerleader, accountability, compassion, and empathy before we can generously give those things to others. I can see you nodding your head saying, *"Yes, it's so much easier to comfort and encourage others and show them grace when they fail, but I don't give myself the same credit, love, or understanding."*

Not giving ourselves enough grace is usually due to:
- A loud inner critic, ego, conditioned self, or small self
- Limiting beliefs
- Our cycles of self-sabotage, criticism, and self-judgment are conditioned
- The way we were raised

- Unresolved pain, wounds, and the past
- We lack understanding around grace and don't have the right tools

We all long for the approval, affection, affirmation, and attention of our parents, friends, kids, and spouse. It isn't wrong, but it isn't healthy when it's a *dependency*, and it determines our state of mind, confidence, decisions, and reactions. Not dealing with our hurts leads to addiction, avoidance, anger, abuse, and the need for approval.

If you can love yourself, compliment yourself, and champion yourself, then you won't be dependent, desperate, or need the validation of others. Of course, we need others and we are made for connection, commitment, and community. Do we thrive on compliments and encouragement? Yes. What I'm saying is many people are dependent on others and have absolutely no dependence on themselves (God and the greatness inside them). If I were to depend on my very quiet husband and children to compliment me daily, I would not be in the best place. So many people place their worth and identity in their relationship status, or other people's approval and affection, and they don't make themselves number one.

Often times, we've had so much pain or abuse growing up (verbal, emotional, physical, or mental), and we are so worried if we don't say "yes" or do "the thing," we will lose the affection, attention, or affirmation of others. Our "yes" is coming from our wounds instead of our true, authentic self. This is what we call a cycle. This cycle will bring pain, disappointment, rejection, disconnection, and loss. There is a way to stop the cycle. It's the power of self.

> **"The foundation of self-love is always forgiveness."**
> — *Dr. Rebecca Ray*

SELF-CARE

"To protect your energy, it's okay to cancel a commitment, not answer a call, change your mind, take time to heal, take a day off, do nothing, speak up, let go, communicate boundaries, share feelings and needs, and take care of you."

Let's talk about self-care, what it is, and how you can begin to implement it into your life. I truly believe being a part of the 5 AM Club and practicing the 20/50/20 method is one of the best things you can do for yourself.

Self-care isn't always beeswax candles and baths, but those are good things, too. Self-care is important. Remember, you always put your oxygen mask on first. Practicing self-care will improve your mood, confidence, peace, positivity, perspective, productivity, and motivation. Being mindful of your habits and thoughts, as well as evaluating your energy and prioritizing self-care, can keep stress down and prevent burnout.

<u>Self-Care Practices</u>:
- Add essential oils to your bath or shower
- Ask for help and delegate
- Boundaries
- Gratitude, gratitude, gratitude
- Write out affirmations, "I Am's," or scriptures
- Write a letter to yourself or a part of you (i.e., mom, spouse)
- Self-compassion
- Read
- Call a friend
- Control what you consume (i.e., If you're sad, don't listen to sad music. If you struggle with fear, don't watch the news or scary shows.)

- Declutter a cabinet, closet, or desk
- Do breathwork (inhale for seven, hold, exhale for seven, repeat) and ground outside
- Eat something healthy
- Go on "field trips"
- Go to a local farm or farmers market and get flowers
- Go to bed early
- Invite friends over for brunch
- Journal
- Look at art
- Make a healthy drink like golden milk or an herbal latte
- Make yourself a nutrient-dense meal and mindfully enjoy it
- Meditate
- Plan a day trip and get something on the calendar you can look forward to
- Practice the 20/50/20 method
- Purchase a new supplement to support your immune system, hormones, stress, or digestive system
- Sit in the sun or sauna for ten to twenty minutes and focus on your breathing
- Schedule regular massages, adjustments, facials, detoxes
- Take a walk in nature
- Take the long way home in silence and appreciate everything you see in nature
- Unplug
- Write a letter (but don't send) of feelings, forgiveness, acceptance, and release to someone who has hurt you

There are many ways to make sure you are taking care of yourself, filling your cup, aligning yourself, healing, growing, and elevating. To neglect self-care would be to miss out on a huge part of wholeness. Without writing a whole book on relationships, it's important to remember we are not dependent on others for our happiness, validation, purpose, healing, or joy.

Our jobs, homes, financial status, and children are not where our hope should lie. For me, my hope is always going to be in God first, then in my relationship with myself. Fun fact, did you know your body knows if you mean what you say? You can speak out all the "good things," but you need to truly believe them, picture them, and trust them more than just say them. I am huge on decrees and affirmations, but the belief is key. The alignment of our thoughts, words, hearts, and actions are what brings true wholeness.

SELF-COMPASSION

> *"If your compassion doesn't include*
> *yourself, it's incomplete."*
> — *Jack Kornfield*

Self-compassion is one of the game-changing tools I have acquired in only the last several years, thanks to Gayle Belanger. I was a born cheerleader of others and myself. I was raised around encouragement, compliments, and faith. I have known about positive self-talk, but self-compassion took it to a new level.

We all have a few voices running through our minds:
1. The ego, inner critic, or conditioned self
2. Our highest self
3. God and the Holy Spirit
4. The enemy

Yes, we can have the voices of those close to us as well (good or bad), but that falls into our conditioned self. Remember, you have the right and power to reject and replace not only your thoughts, ego, and the enemy's voice, but other people's negative voices or word curses.

The word *compassion* means sympathetic concern for the sufferings or misfortunes of others. If we are in tune with our mind, body, and spirit, and living from a healthy place, we typically can extend and feel compassion for others. It might be for a person in a wheelchair at the grocery store, the child being yelled at by his mother in a store, the homeless person on your local corner, a friend who lost their job, and so on. When you see a baby learning to walk and they fall, do you criticize and yell at them to get back up? No. They are learning, they are growing, they are in process.

So often we treat our healing, growth, feelings, and situations with such criticism and unrealistic pressures. Would we do that to a friend or our own child? Yes and no. Are there times we are very critical of others? Yes. The more critical we are of others, and the less compassion and empathy we feel for others is only a reflection of our inner world. Those who hurt others the most are hurting the most inside. There are many times we can be quick to acknowledge, praise, comfort, and encourage others even in their mistakes, but we would not think to give that same love to ourselves.

Self-compassion is offering understanding and kindness to oneself. For example, instead of shoving, ignoring, and repressing hard or hurtful things, you can stop and say, "Wow this is hard, and I know this doesn't feel good, but it is going to be okay." When you spill something or make a simple mistake, the voice of our critic says, "You're so stupid. You're dumb. Why did you do that? Do you ever learn? What a joke." Or it loves to tell us, "That won't work out. They don't love you. You're ugly. You will never measure up." This, my friends, is self-criticism and the polar opposite of self-compassion.

When we realize that failure, hurt, mistakes, and pain are all part of humanity, we can extend deeper empathy to ourselves and others. We are all experiencing something. Honoring, accepting, and acknowledging are all acts of self-compassion. This doesn't mean you will never have a harsh thought or response again, but it means they will become less or only last a few moments. Then you can transmute those thoughts and feelings through a filter of love, acceptance, acknowledgment, and comfort. No one is on a perfect streak in life and winning in all areas; we are all learning, healing, growing, and processing.

> **"If you don't love yourself, you can't love others.**
> **If you have no compassion for yourself,**
> **then you are not able of developing**
> **compassion for others."**
> — *Dalai Lama*

One of the greatest benefits of self-compassion I have found is that my need to go to others for validation, empathy, and acceptance (which they often can't offer as well as I expect, especially as a "words" gal) can now be met within myself. I am my own biggest fan, encouragement, and empathy.

When my teenagers say hurtful things, I can have healthy boundaries with them, communicate with *I feel* and *I need* statements, and set standards of communication. Next, I have instant self-compassion that looks something like this: (speaking to the mother part of me) *Wow, that was so hard to hear, that was so hurtful. Wow, he was just mean. Ouch. I can see how that was a low blow, and you didn't deserve that. I am so sorry he said that. Those words are not true. You are a great mom.* I then forgive and release.

This point is a great time to apply the RRRR tool I shared in *The Power of Peace, Love, and Gratitude,* and to also forgive, release, and surrender the hurt, the words, and the exchange. I have practiced this with mean customers, haters on the internet, and exchanges with family or friends. I have also used it when I have been out of line, judgmental, sassy, messed something up, had a negative mindset, or forgot something. Shame, guilt, and regret are such destiny and greatness robbers. If only we would extend compassion, forgiveness, and grace, so much self-hate could be prevented.

There are a few ways we can practice self-compassion, but the key is really to talk and respond to yourself or your situation as you would a good friend. Just touching your own hand, breathing through a conversation, or self-regulating your thoughts and emotions can help.

The other part is not only using this tool in low moments, but also celebrating your daily wins, growth, and progress. Give yourself *that-a-girl* or *that-a-boy* high-fives, so to say. This is really important. When you find old situations no longer trigger you, people's approval no longer rules you, insecurities no longer haunt you, and pain no longer consumes you, it is important to recognize, honor, and celebrate.

Please understand many people aren't able to give love, kindness, empathy, grace, and compassion. They might not have been raised with or been taught how, and their repressed pain and self-criticism prevents them from loving you and loving themselves. Please choose to have compassion for where they are instead of judgment, and understand it's not about you.

> *"Do not allow any outside circumstance to be more powerful than your internal world."*
> — *Unknown*

A STEP FURTHER

> *"If outside validation is your only source of nourishment, you will hunger for the rest of your life."*
> — *Unknown*

I am going to share something very personal and vulnerable to me, so please take great care of my heart. This is for those of us who have a relationship (not religion or legalism) with God, Jesus, and the Holy Spirit, and believe in our eternal and true self. We can bring these parts into our self-compassion. Now, we are not only getting empathy, kindness, validation, and acceptance from ourselves, but also God.

This is a huge part of our relationship with Him—He is our source of truth, comfort, love, validation and beyond. I'm not looking for my kids, my spouse, my work, or my gifts to bring those to my life; they are bonuses and blessings. I find those in Him. I'm not putting pressure on everyone around me to meet my needs, encourage, and comfort me all the time because I'm getting that in the practices found in these powerful sections, as well as from Jesus.

As believers, we know we are seated at the right hand of God, and there is our eternal person who has no pain, sin, sickness, doubt, or fear. Again, we often need to ask our thoughts, emotions, and words, "What voice is this?" and know that if it is not full of hope, love, empathy, and peace, then it's coming from our pain, ego, or the enemy.

It's time to change the channel. You can visualize sitting on a park bench or being on a sports field, or wherever your special place with God is in your mind, eyes, and imagination, and know you can go to that place at any time for peace, truth, comfort, healing, hope, and wisdom. I check on all the parts of me almost daily. Remember, we are not just mom, wife, business owner, or builder—those are only hats and roles we play.

I will check in on my mom self, business owner self, friend self, and daughter self to see if certain parts of me need hope, healing, love, or compassion. These practices have helped me not only heal, but get out of a funk, self-pity, pain, projection, blame, and so much more. I'm able to see, feel, and hear what's going on and tend to that part with God.

It might look like (in my spiritual imagination) getting a hug, having Jesus make me a special tea and tell me about how it's healing my jaded heart, renewing my broken mind, inspiring good within me, or hearing all the words I long to hear from those around me. Remember, friends, happiness is an inside job. We are not to depend on others, things, or circumstances to make us happy; they are only added blessings to our already happy, aligned, centered, and internal world.

There might be times the pain is so great, and a part of us is hurting or grieving so much we will need to give ourselves time and space. Grieving is healthy and a process. Grief is not only for physical death, but for the death of relationships, dreams, ideas, perceptions, and attachments. There are full books written in depths on all of this, and I am only giving you the basics to help you start your very own self-compassion practice. If you are a believer, hopefully this helps spark a new element of your relationship with God. He loves to partner with us, always has time for us, is always for us, and will never leave us, forsake us, or hurt us.

I acknowledge and understand this may seem crazy, intense, woo woo, or impossible to you. I also get that many people have a complicated relationship and view of God. Know that anything is possible, every day is a new day, and no past, person, force, heart, mind, situation, or pain is greater than love.

CHAPTER TEN

NEXT LEVEL LIVING

"Ordinary people love leisure; icons love learning."

This place in the book is a great grounding point and reference to be shared with the masses. Let's call this the summary or CliffsNotes version of *Healing Through Wisdom*. If you wanted to help someone take some fast action, you could take a photo of this and send it to them. The "how-tos" are shared in detail through many chapters of this book, but sometimes we need to see things over and over to really let them soak into our mind, body, and spirit. These are principles I have taught, used, and shared for years.

Ten Keys to Wholeness:
1. Positivity
2. Purpose: *love, care, serve*
3. Gratitude
4. People and community: *have coaches and mentors*
5. Faith and belief
6. Mindsets and identity

7. Education and personal growth
8. Physical health: *sleep, hydration, exercise, supplements, eating clean, non-toxic home and hygiene, regular detoxing (see my holistic practices in* Holistic Must-Haves and Pantry Swaps)
9. Daily practices and disciplines: *meditation, 20/50/20 morning routine, self-compassion, heal, forgive*
10. Management: *yourself, your money and resources, your health, your time, and your relationships*

<u>Practices of Next Level Living:</u>

- Always learn.
- Always forgive.
- Be healthy in your communication (i.e., I feel, I need), including healthy confrontation.
- Develop excellent time management and boundaries.
- Keep a clear "why."
- Keep a humble heart and a positive mind.
- Have the right people on the bus and in the circle.
- Make health a priority.
- Never repress emotions or feelings.
- Practice compassion (self and others); care deeply.
- Pray and meditate.
- Stay accountable and submitted.

Now, we know a list is only as powerful as the application. These are very effective core laws and commandments of next level living. If you're reading this book, it's because you want to live well, be whole, and find breakthrough. You want to fulfill your purpose, you want to have an epic life, you want to impact the world around you, and you want to leave a legacy. It's going to take grit, grind, and grace. I know you have it in you. I know you have wells of love, determination, hope, and passion ready to pour out.

CHAPTER ELEVEN

WISDOM SAYS

"Where there is wisdom, there is always hope.
Wisdom simplifies. Wisdom clarifies.
Wisdom untangles. Wisdom unshackles.
Wisdom illuminates."
— *Erwin McManus*

I think it's important to clarify what exactly wisdom is and what wisdom has to say about health and healing.

Wisdom says everything is a choice.
Wisdom says no one is responsible for your health but you.
Wisdom says your genes are not your destiny.
Wisdom says not to wait, and not to put off what you know needs to happen now.
Wisdom says that when you know better, you do better.
Wisdom says to do what's right, not what's convenient.
Wisdom says to read ingredients and labels.
Wisdom says fuel, not food.
Wisdom says if it's on a commercial, don't eat it, buy it, or use it.

Wisdom says to get your blood work done, get allergy tested, and get your hormone panel done.

Wisdom says to find out what is most effective for you, not what a book says.

Wisdom says to try things for at least ninety consistent days.

Wisdom says if a specific thing isn't working for you, try another thing.

Wisdom says it's a practice and a process, and change won't happen overnight; trust the process.

Wisdom says not to quit.

Wisdom says shortcuts don't always pay off.

Wisdom says when you mess up and get off track, start again.

Wisdom says compromise never feels good in the end.

Wisdom says to trust your gut.

Wisdom says no one wins, heals, or changes alone, and to choose community over everything.

Wisdom says to seek wise counsel and that in the counsel of many, you will succeed.

Wisdom says to find people and a tribe who are like-minded so you can be on this journey together.

Wisdom says surround yourself with people who care, see you, and deploy empathy and greatness.

Wisdom says not to be a sheeple.

Wisdom says discipline is gritty, rewarding, and not easy but necessary.

Wisdom says never settle and never stop learning.

Wisdom says you must apply knowledge to see its benefit.

Wisdom says to ask questions.

Wisdom says to get a second and third opinion.

Wisdom says to get a new provider if your current one doesn't support or practice functional medicine.

Wisdom says there are other options besides procedures, chemo, and prescriptions.

Wisdom says to see a holistic nutritionist.

Wisdom says not to expect a non-expert to go deep into blood work or hormone panels.

Wisdom says alternative health and Eastern medicine are not "hocus pocus."

Wisdom says preventative healthcare is wise.

Wisdom says not to wait to take vitamins until you're over thirty.

Wisdom says it's better to be called a hippie than unhealthy.

Wisdom says to ignore the critics.

Wisdom says fluoride is not your friend.

Wisdom says choose well, live well, love well, and be well.

Wisdom says those aren't clouds; those are chemtrails.

Wisdom says the sun is not Satan, but organic sunblock is wise after an hour.

Wisdom says to measure success by the state of your mindset, heartset, healthset, and spiritset.

Wisdom says to fight for your health, your healing, and your future.

Wisdom says to forgive; bitterness is poison.

Wisdom says to reject every lie, limiting belief, and word curse.

Wisdom says comfortable is another word for complacent.

Wisdom says not to expect health when you are speaking death.

Wisdom says to laugh, smile, and celebrate.

Wisdom says to know your worth and be a person of value.

Wisdom says loving yourself is not selfish; it's sacred.

"Wisdom says wisdom is better than strength."
— *King Solomon*

CHAPTER TWELVE

IT MATTERS

WHEN YOU HAVE HEALTH, YOU HAVE EVERYTHING

"Faith is necessary, patience is key,
discipline is everything, focus is priority,
and execution is mandatory."

You have peace. You have energy. You have clarity. You have stamina. You have creativity. You have strength. You have hope. You have possibility. You have opportunity. You have happiness. You have movement. You have perspective. You have rest. You have choices. You have harmony. You have sustainability. You have heroism.

For the record, I have seen people with health challenges have better attitudes, mindsets, passion, and hope than those with "full health." Health is so many things: Physical. Mental. Emotional. Spiritual. Relational. Financial. Community. Purpose.

This past Christmas, I kept thinking how the greatest gifts are not just to have faith, friends, and family, but that those friends and family are present, they are with us, they are healthy, they are capable, and they are safe. These are the treasures of life: to fully live, be fully alive, and to be with loved ones.

Never take for granted the health you have. If you are sleeping, have energy, have a clear mind, and not on medication, you are one of the rare ones. The things becoming sadly normal in our society are sickness, disease, depression, and brokenness. I know this is not what was intended for our brilliant and beautiful souls.

If you don't have your health, what do you have at the end of the day? Nothing else holds as much weight as your health. I realize there are many people doing amazing things who have physical limitations, but their mindset is much stronger than their circumstances. This is why the focus has to be *mind, body, and spirit*.

I am seriously inspired by those who are physically limited, like Inky Johnson and Nick Vujicic. They are proof of what the mind is capable of and what the Spirit is capable of with work, healing, and hope. Icons like Nelson Mandela, Martin Luther, Cyrus, Chief Joseph, Rosa Parks, and Viktor Frankl are a few who also come to mind. They faced incredible opposition, culture wars, hate, and so much more, but they had incredible mindsets, resilience, and are an example of being a heroic icon. Their mindsets helped them overcome impossible odds.

We all have a legend inside of us who wants to fulfill the God-given calling, but health must be aligned and boundaries and systems must in place, or we may find an early death, burnout, or breakdowns. At the end of the day, we all want to sleep well, feel good, think clearly, have hopeful hearts, good relationships, a strong foundation, believe, trust, and have the energy to complete our personal tasks, our work tasks, and our purpose.

Have you ever played a game like Taboo or a fast-paced guessing game, with a diverse age range of people? It is said that the younger players do better because their neurons are firing faster and on all cylinders. This might be true, but some of it could be a personal choice. We have a cellular age and our numerical age. You can see living proof on people's faces with this.

I actually know people in their thirties who are not as healthy as some people in their fifties, and their energy levels don't even compare. It isn't just about age; it's about maintenance. It's about mindset, emotional health, and daily choices.

You don't have to have cancer or be in a hospital bed to be "unhealthy." I talk at length in this book about the emotional, mental, personal, and spiritual sides of health. They can't be ignored, and if they are, it's only so long until they show up on your doorstep.

It can be hard at times to hear people talk about chronic pain, chronic discomfort, chronic digestive issues, headaches, fatigue, and sleep issues, yet they're not willing to look at their diet, the medications they're taking, or the products they're using day in and day out. All of this could very well be resolved not by a pill, but by wisdom and diligence.

High-performing athletes are usually in tune with their bodies as they want to perform well, which means they must practice well and recover well. Even just a small headache or a slightly stuffy nose can affect their energy or performance, though many legends have powered through. Take Michael Jordon for example. He played while fighting the flu and still hit insane numbers. Because of this, Nike released a shoe called *'Flu Game*. Talk about mindset, willpower, and drive!

For many people, health is keeping them from their best life, slowing them down, and forcing them to say *no* when they would like to say *yes*. They are not bringing their A-game. We have to grasp how important our bodies actually are, how important our mindset is, and how important it is to not poison ourselves with apathy, criticism, unforgiveness, and bitterness.

We don't fill our homes with chemicals, slather our bodies with toxins, feed our bodies fake foods, and fill our minds with pointless entertainment and still call it a life. We don't numb our feelings, silence our voices, ignore our greatness, repress our pain, and speak horribly to ourselves only to believe the lies and live at a low frequency. Your "health bank account" is keeping a record even when you're not. It is digesting what you're depositing, and it is giving you only what it has. It might not go so well if you try to withdraw peace of mind, strong immunity, and clarity when all you put in is negativity and Taco Bell. Actually, we know for sure it won't.

A question I'm often asked or overhear people saying is, *"Does it even matter? At the end of the day, at the end of my life, does it actually matter?"* As you've read this far, you might be saying, *"Chrissy, I hear what you're saying, and I want to make all the changes and do all the things, but does it really matter that much? Is it really worth it?"* To you, my friend, I say keep on reading.

DOES IT MATTER?

I often find the things prohibiting people from pursuing true health are lies, limiting beliefs, or self-sabotage. The most common one is *Does it really matter?*

Does it really matter if I eat GMO?
Does it really matter if I pray, meditate, and exercise?
Do my thoughts really matter?
Do my words really matter?
Is any of this actually doing anything?
Does organic even mean anything?
Do vitamins matter?
If everything is so bad, then it doesn't really matter what I do? I'm going to die anyway. *(Well, you only live once, so you may as well enjoy it.)*
If I'm going down, at least I'll go down eating what I want to eat. *(Shout-out to my sister and her churros!)*
If we weren't supposed to eat this, then it wouldn't be available.

I would suggest you go back to the first time you started to think that way, or maybe the first time something didn't go as planned. It's important to be healed from those things so you no longer sabotage the effort you put forth, or try to convince yourself it doesn't matter and end up justified doing whatever you want.

This is especially true for people who called themselves a leader or believer and think there is some magical prayer, mantra, or wand that's going to take chemicals out of food or there's a blessing on knowingly putting toxic things into their bodies. That is a scary practice. As Christians, I think we're really quick to bless it and a little too slow to actually research it—whether that be our food, medications, treatments, toxic cleaners, lotions, or air fresheners. This isn't just a believer thing or Christian thing. Yes, a lot of this is a humanity thing, but I do feel the need to speak to those of the faith, as I believe we have a calling to raise the standard, be set apart, and steward well.

I totally get that if you don't know what's in your food or in the product you're using, there is grace on that. But once we know better, we do better. I believe, just as many people who experience spiritual transformation and awakening, we can also have the same type of awakening with health where it's no longer about *maybe I should,* or *maybe I shouldn't,* but it becomes a conviction. Especially if you have a high call and purpose on your life and you want to honor the greatness, gifts, icon, and hero inside of you.

Your health decisions are not just affecting you. We all want to live the longest, strongest, and best quality of life possible, as well as help those in our lives and those who might be taking care of us in the future. How is it fair for our children to need to take care of us at a young, "old age" because we didn't make better choices along the way? When you say it doesn't matter, how do you think that would make your spouse feel, your parents feel, or your children feel? Do you want to put the burden on them to take care of you or to worry about you because you didn't take care of yourself? We already know this is the reality for many.

Children watch our every move, including choosing between TV and reading; they replicate what they see. If you drive through Taco Bell, they are likely to drive through Taco Bell. Yes, that can be changed, as people have their own inner-compass and convictions. I'm living proof of doing things differently, and the changes I've made along the way have affected my family for the better.

Now, I want to shatter the above lies and limiting beliefs with something mind-blowing. Are you ready for it?

IT DOES MATTER

I think teenagers are probably some of the most guilty for saying things like, "I don't care. Whatever. It doesn't matter," as it pertains to a lot more things than phones. Try telling a teenager how social media, EMFs, blue light, and technology really affects them and let me know how that turns out for you. Try telling them how important it is to floss, forgive, have self-compassion, or communicate in a healthy way. Good luck, yet don't give up.

Maybe the translation there actually is: *This is really hard. I don't have the support that I need. I don't know where to start. I'm afraid to fail. I'm scared. What if they _____. I'm scared of not fitting in. I don't know how to stop _____. I'm afraid of getting hurt. I'm believing lies. My mind is saying I'm not worthy of the investment or the effort.*

This, my friends, is where we must begin. Start with feeling and revealing those lies so that we can get them out of the way. Change your belief system and change your thoughts (as I taught you to in *The Power of Self*) so we can maximize the decisions we're making for our mental, spiritual, and emotional health.

People you love will continue to make choices that cause you to cringe and cry, and you can only do so much. Share the "whys" in love, plant seeds, and let it go. I have told my teenagers so many times, "If you really love yourself and did things considering your future self, then your decisions may look different." Eating a bunch of Sour Patch Kids is not really in alignment with health; you are either feeding health or feeding sickness with every thought and every bite.

It is so important to be aware on every level from our thoughts to our food, from what alternatives we have to certain modern treatments, and from what we brush our teeth with to what we slather on our bodies. Awareness gives you the opportunity to make a different decision. When we research and empower ourselves with alternatives and options, we are less likely to make emotional decisions or misguided choices regarding our health. Yes, we want to trust, but we also want to use wisdom, care, and truth to guide the decisions affecting our homes, earth, health, and futures.

> *"We can't solve our problems with the same*
> *thinking we used when we created them."*
> — *Albert Einstein*

I cannot say it enough: *This stuff matters!* It matters for our communities and our earth. Can you imagine what all the narcotic waste and toxic food waste is doing to our planet? I'm sure someone's written a book on this alone. It's doing incredible damage as far as mental health goes, that's for sure. The system has us where they want us—*numb and dumb*. Won't you revolt with me? Many children and adults are misdiagnosed with ADHD, bipolar, or other things, when really they are allergic, intolerant, or sensitive to certain types of foods, and they are deficient in some core essentials.

Instead of only choosing pills or procedures, we can choose effective alternatives. When our communities are healthy, we are involved. We are active, we are present, we are powerful. When the earth is healthy, we are not only stewarding well but adding value to our planet and the future. We are responsible for more of the earth's condition than we give ourselves credit for. Healthy choices lead to healthy people. Healthy people lead to healthy families. And healthy families lead to healthy communities and healthy futures.

Let's reject and replace these lies, assumptions, excuses, and distractions from greatness. Here are some of the lies keeping us from doing better and owning the fact that *it matters:*

- I've always lived this way, and I'm fine.
- Everyone I know is fine. (Not possible.)
- It doesn't matter.
- It's too expensive.
- I don't have time.
- I don't know what to do.
- It's not that bad.
- If it is so bad, why does everyone live this way?
- I'll always be healthy.
- So-and-so didn't, and they lived a long time.
- _____ (symptom) isn't a big deal.
- No awareness of health at any level to even know or recognize something is on or off (living numb and dumb).
- If _____ were so bad, it wouldn't be legal, and so many people wouldn't enjoy it.
- I have lots of time to make changes and get healthy.
- I know it's bad for me, but I don't care.
- I know its bad for me, but I can't X-Y-Z (victim mindset).
- It's too expensive (scarcity mindset).
- The world will end any moment anyway, so why care?

I know these are not the only lies that allow us to swim in pools of *it doesn't matter*, but it's a great start for punching them in the face and taking ownership of our futures. Remember, we are powerful, wise, capable, and amazing co-creators. Nothing is impossible with wisdom, willpower, strategy, dedication, community, and execution. Let's resist the passivity, excuses, and empty promises to our self and others and begin to take one step, one action, one day at a time.

"Discipline and desire go hand-in-hand. Whatever you desire is where you must discipline yourself the most. Sacrifice always accompanies discipline."

CHAPTER THIRTEEN

WHERE DO I START?

Friends, well done! Reading up to this point is a huge accomplishment, and I acknowledge that you stuck with it. You've allowed it to speak to every part of you, not just your mind. Maybe now you're seeing and believing how your health is everything, and you want to take action to heal your mind, body, and spirit, as well as improve your life, create a legacy, and walk in your purpose. I'm so here for it!

Considering we covered a lot of territory, you will need to decide what the top priority is for you and your health. There are things you can start right away that don't cost a dime or take much effort. Some of those are journaling, self-regulating your thoughts, meditation, working out, waking up earlier, tossing out some toxic products, and getting better sleep. You might already know and live some of what's been shared, so now is the time to take the new parts and execute to the next level. The keys to this book are application, consistency, accountability, and execution.

A few other things to consider would be:
- Deeper steps, like blood work, a detox, gut healing, metal detox, a cleanse, a home detox, diet change, a trainer, thera-

pist, and/or life coach.
- Focus on what you can do right now with what you have and where you're at.
- Get connected to all of the great resources, blogs, podcasts, natural-minded practitioners, and community in your local area.
- Head to the *Healing Through Wisdom* Facebook group.
- Identify and treat any "silent enemies."
- Identify the lies, cycles, and sabotages that have kept you from your best.
- Share the truths in this book. Start now with at least one other person.
- Sign up for Thrive Market and Butcher Box.

It will be important for you to get on some kind of protocol and have the right things under your sink, in your pantry, and "medicine" cabinet so you are set up for success. Again, every person is different based on blood type, nutrition needs, conditions, and age. I can only give a blanket and general guide for what typically works as a good baseline for most people. I passionately believe in partnering with the right healthcare team for your success. In the following chapter, I give detailed resources, like holistic checklists, pantry swap tips, and home remedies.

Basic Keys to Health:
- Avoid chemicals in your home (cleaning products, hygiene products, pesticides).
- Be in community.
- Drink water (half your body weight in ounces).
- Eat clean. This includes your water.
- Exercise twenty to sixty minutes per day. Sweating is essential to health.
- Get sunshine and fresh air.
- Get the best sleep possible.
- Guard your heart, thoughts, and your words, as well as train

and heal them.
- Limit EMF exposure.
- Meditate, pray, and journal.
- Serve, give, and care.
- Take core supplements: probiotics, D3, magnesium.

Clean Eating: The easiest way to understand clean eating is that it's eating real food in its least processed form. You should be able to pronounce and recognize every ingredient and know what type of plant it came from. It should be "nature-made" as much as possible and have real nutrients (additives and preservatives are a *no*). Remember, labels and branding mean nothing; ingredients mean everything. Count chemicals, not calories. Clean eating is mindful eating. You can enjoy tons of delicious and filling foods when you eat clean. You want to make sure your food is organic as much as possible, as well as avoid refined and processed sugar (yes, even organic sugar is still refined sugar), grains, flours, and conventional animal products (meat, eggs, dairy). This is not a diet but a lifestyle.

FRUITS *(organic)*

Apples	Nectarines
Avocado	Oranges
Bananas	Peaches
Berries	Pears
Cherries	Pineapple
Dates	Plantains
Figs	Plums
Grapes	Pomegranate
Kiwi	Watermelon
Mango	
Melon	

FATS AND OILS *(organic)*

Avocado oil
Beef tallow (grass-fed)
Coconut oil
Duck fat
Ghee (grass-fed)
Lard
Olive oil
Raw butter (grass-fed)
Sesame oil

VEGETABLES *(organic)*

Acorn squash
Artichoke
Arugula
Asparagus
Beets
Bell pepper
Bok choy
Broccoli
Brussels sprouts
Butternut squash
Cabbage
Carrots
Cauliflower
Celery
Collard greens
Cucumber
Eggplant
Fennel
Green beans
Kale
Leek
Lettuce
Mushrooms
Onion
Parsnips
Pea sprouts
Potatoes
Spinach
Sprouts
Squash
Sweet potatoes/yams
Swiss chard
Tomato
Zucchini

PROTEINS *(organic, pasture-raised, grass-fed and -finished, nitrate-free and/or wild-caught)*

Beef
Bison
Chicken
Deli meat
Duck
Eggs
Fish
Lamb
Pork
Turkey

NUTS AND SEEDS *(organic and mold-free)*

Almonds
Brazil nuts
Cashews
Chia seeds
Flax seeds
Hazelnuts
Macadamia nuts
Pecans
Pine nuts
Pistachios
Pumpkin seeds/pepitas
Sesame seeds
Sunflower seeds
Walnuts

OTHER PROTEINS *(organic)*

Black beans
Certain raw cheeses
Kefir
Lentils

This is a great start for you to know what you can and get to enjoy. Healthy living is never about deprivation, but celebration. Your "why" and your knowledge of the truth will drive you to choose well—once you break free from your sugar addiction, that is. You can do it!

I encourage you to find what works for your season of life—be that paleo, primal paleo, paleotarian (as Dr. Hyman would call it), Whole30, keto, or clean. I only ask that it's organic and clean. You will find real food tastes *real* and actually leaves you full. How amazing is that? You can also find amazing meal plans, meal deliveries, and health coaches to help you on this journey. Cheers to eating well and feeling better!

CHAPTER FOURTEEN

HOLISTIC MUST-HAVES AND PANTRY SWAPS

I have mentioned throughout the book the foundational supplements for all ages are magnesium, probiotics, and vitamin D3. This chapter is devoted to giving you holistic, nature-based remedies and key supports for optimal health. I'll suggest holistic alternatives for the top health concerns people come into my store with daily. Before listing all these supports though, it is important to describe why the three foundational supplements are non-negotiable.

> **"Many people are waiting on a miracle**
> **when really they just need magnesium."**

Magnesium is the fourth most abundant mineral in the body, right next to sulfur (which is just as important). It is *everything*. People press that we need water and air, yet skip over this essential mineral we all desperately need. Did you know you need magnesium to *live*? Without electrolytes like magnesium, your muscles can't fire, your heart can't beat, and your brain can't receive signals. Many functional medicine and holistic practitioners will tell you that every issue or disease is tied to a magnesium deficiency. Anything that makes you tense and tight could potentially be caused by a magnesium deficiency. If you can't relax or you can't stop—think magnesium! Full-blown health problems can even be tied back to this crucial mineral. Insane, right? Curious why we have this magnesium crisis? I believe it's because we are being poisoned slowly with many of the things talked about this in this book (foods, refined sugars, toxins, and our environment). Even if you eat kale and drink wheatgrass all day, you still *need* magnesium. I suggest using both magnesium citrate (Trace Minerals or Garden of Life brands), along with a magnesium oil *spray* (Trace Minerals) on the bottom of your feet every night for the best absorption.

Probiotics are essential to gut health. They are healthy cultures and bacteria that our digestive system, brain, and gut needs. Digestive experts agree that the balance of gut flora should be approximately 85 percent good bacteria and 15 percent bad bacteria. As I mentioned earlier, our gut and brain are connected, so ensuring our gut is in line and healthy is key for ideal brain function. A healthy gut is a healthy brain and mind. Probiotics should be taken daily for optimal health. Also, a major key with probiotics is they are not all created equal. You want to get the ones that are food-based or kept in the fridge, such as The Coconut Cult (dairy-, gluten-, soy-, and sugar-free), fermented foods (if you're not battling candida, SIBO, or parasites), or in supplement form with a range from fifteen billion to one hundred billion strains. If you are healing your gut or working on your GI, you will want to take the highest amount and quality possible. Probiotics are necessary for all ages, considering over 70 percent of the immune system is in the gut. Remember, our gut is our second brain, so we need to be feeding and supporting it with quality probiotics.

Vitamin D3 is something we typically get from the sun, but sadly, the sun is no longer what it used to be due to environmental toxins. We also are inside more than ever before, so we lack this essential nutrient. Vitamin D3 is not only good for mood, sleep, and immunity, but it's also connected to heart health. Checking D3 levels is pretty mainstream now, even in Western medicine, and most people are very low in D3; studies show 90 percent of people are deficient. You can get D3 in supplements and foods, such as raw dairy and fermented cod liver oil, and sunshine (ideally between 10:00 AM and 3:00 PM). Often, just adding vitamin D3, probiotics, and magnesium can change the status of your health far more than you would expect if you are generally healthy.

> *"I've got ninety-nine problems,*
> *but healing my gut solved almost all of them."*

HOLISTIC MUST-HAVES

Supplements 101:
- Activated charcoal
- Adrenal support (ashwagandha and holy basil)
- B-complex
- Bee propolis
- Brain Octane Oil
- Camu camu
- Chlorophyll
- Chlorella
- Collagen
- Colloidal silver
- Essential oils
- Fermented cod liver oil
- Fire Cider
- Garden of Life
- Grape seed extract (GSE)
- Maca root with selenium
- Magnesium

- Manuka honey 13+
- Multi-mushroom blend
- Nootropics
- N-acetyl cysteine (NAC)
- Probiotics
- Raw vitamin C
- Revive Multi
- Silica
- Spirulina
- Superfood blend
- Vital Proteins
- Vitamin D3

PANTRY SWAPS

THIS	NOT THAT
Grass-fed, raw butter or ghee	Conventional butter
Unreal and Hu chocolate	Justin's chocolate candy
Nut, goat, or raw cheese	American cheese
Siete tortilla chips	Tostitos
Raw, nut, or oat milk	Fat-free, lactose-free, or 1% milk
Almond, sprouted spelt, coconut, or cassava flour	Bleached wheat flour
Fermented, organic sourdough	Oroweat or Wonder Bread
Coconut, olive, or avocado oil	Crisco, canola, or vegetable oil
Grass-fed and -finished meat	Natural or conventional meat
Sprouted brown basmati rice	White rice
Primal Kitchen or homemade salad dressing	Ranch or store-bought salad dressing
Coconut aminos	Tamari or regular soy sauce
Monk fuit, coconut sugar, maple syrup, or honey	Refined sugars

HOUSEHOLD SWAPS

THIS	NOT THAT
Bamboo, silk, linen, or cotton	Synthetic materials
Beeswax candles	Soy or paraffin wax candles
Buy in bulk/refill containers	Buy new in new packaging
Eco-friendly soaps and cleaners	Conventional cleaners
Essential oils	Fragrance and air fresheners
Vinegar and lemon	Bleach
Washcloths	Cotton rounds
Norwex cleaning cloths	Bleached paper towels
Avocado/Naturepedic mattress	Chemical, synthetic foam mattress
Berkey filtered water	Brita filtered water
Biokleen Back-Out or Stain Stick	Tide to Go
Grocery shop with resuable bags	Plastic shopping and produce bags
Donate	Accumulate
Glass	Plastic
Resuable metal or paper straws	Plastic straws
Silverware or compostable cutlery	Plastic, one-time-use cutlery
Reusable food wraps	Single-use
Dryer balls	Dryer sheets
Convection oven	Microwave
Secondhand and/or fair trade	Fast fashion
Eco-friendly baking paper	Aluminum foil
Bath ball and shower filter	Chlorinated city shower water
Compost	Throwing food into landfills
Salt lamps	Night lights
Airplane mode	Keeping WiFi and Bluetooth on
Quality air filters	Ineffective and bleached filters

REMEDIES AND SUPPORTS

Allergy Remedies:
- Air filters
- Allergy Blend by Gaia
- Bee pollen
- Daily celery juice in the morning
- Elderberry
- Whole World Royal Desmodium
- Lavender essential oil
- Lemon essential oil
- Peppermint essential oil
- Raw dairy
- Raw local honey
- Respiratory blend essential oil
- Salt lamps

Baby Reflux Remedies:
- Baltic Amber or Hazelwood necklace
- Chiropractor
- Digestive Blend essential oil on tummy before each feeding
- Elimination diet (if you're breastfeeding, try the FODMAP diet)
- Feed with baby's head propped up
- Massage
- Probiotics
- Upright for thirty minutes after feeding
- Use an organic, pure formula without sugar, gluten, or corn if breastmilk is not an option. Other alternatives are donor milk or follow the Weston A. Price recipe.

Combat Colds for Little Ones:
- Breastfeed
- Chiropractor
- Colloidal silver

- Echinacea (alcohol-free), one drop per two pounds they weigh
- Elderberry syrup (one year and older)
- Grape seed extract
- Colloidal silver
- Nose Frida
- Probiotics (rub on gums or put into a liquid)
- Propolis and apple cider vinegar in smoothie (one year and up)
- Respiratory blend, On Guard, or melaleuca essential oils (topically and in diffuser or humidifier)
- Sleep propped up
- Vitamin D3 and vitamin C

Cough and Sore Throat Remedies:
- Bone Broth
- Bronchial Wellness by Gaia
- Colloidal silver
- Echinacea Goldenseal Propolis throat spray by Gaia
- Elderberry syrup
- Gargle melaleuca and Himalayan salt or silver
- Herbal blend lung support
- Pineapple juice
- Propolis capsules and propolis paste
- Raw honey and raw Manuka honey 13+
- Respiratory oils
- Throat Coat tea
- Wellness Tea (see recipe on page 255)

Detox List:
- Activated charcoal
- Alpha lipoic acids (i.e., Brussels sprouts, broccoli, spinach)
- Bentonite clay
- Bone broth
- Chelation therapy
- Chlorella

- Cilantro
- Citrus fruits
- Coffee enemas
- Curcumin (Bulletproof brand)
- Detox baths: Epsom salt, vitamin C powder, bentonite clay, CBD (THC-free)
- Detox smoothies
- Garlic
- Ginger
- Glutathione
- High doses of vitamin C
- Massage and lymphatic drainage
- Milk thistle
- Probiotics
- Selenium
- Shilajit
- Spirulina
- TRS spray

Digestive Tips:
- Activated charcoal
- Amino acids
- Avoid grains, conventional animal products, and processed food
- CBD (THC-free)
- Chew slowly and eat consciously
- Chiropractor and exercise
- Daily probiotics
- Digestive Blend essential oil
- Digestive enzymes
- Fermented foods
- Gut healing and detox
- No drinks with meal, only before or after
- Raw dairy (specifically kefir)
- Intermittent fasting

Ear Infection or Earache Remedies:

- Basil oil and melaleuca oil rubbed behind ear with carrier oil. Put on cotton ball, then cotton ball in ear.
- Colloidal silver
- Ear candling and ear adjustments
- Garlic oil (see recipe below)
- Immune supports

Garlic oil works amazingly well to kill ear infections, but fresh garlic is best. When garlic is chopped and pressed, the compound alliin converts to allicin, which is the compound responsible for garlic's amazing powers. Not only does the garlic need to be chopped for this conversion to happen, but after about an hour, it starts to degrade to the point that it is rendered ineffective. This is why garlic pills are such a sham. Making your own garlic oil is easy and quick.

Recipe:

1/4 cup extra-virgin olive oil
4-5 cloves of garlic
2-4 drops per ear

Chop 4-5 cloves and let sit 10 minutes. Meanwhile, warm extra-virgin olive oil over very low heat (you just want to warm it). Pour over chopped garlic and let sit 15-60 minutes. Strain out garlic chunks and transfer garlic-infused oil into a glass jar. Administer 2-4 drops using a medicine dropper into the ear canal every hour. Warm oil before each use by placing the jar in a bowl of hot water. Place a warm rice sock (salt sock is even better) on affected ear. Warmth really helps, so be sure to warm the oil and use the compress. This usually kills the infection after only one or two doses and offers immediate relief from the pain associated with the infection.

<u>Energy and Focus Boosters:</u>
- Brain Octane Oil (Bulletproof)
- Chlorella
- Fire Cider
- Hydrate (water, coconut water with lemon and chia seeds)
- Nootropics
- Peppermint oil (drop in palm of hands, rub together, inhale deeply)
- Raw apple cider vinegar
- Shot of chlorophyll to your water daily, in a juice, or on its own
- Superfood blend (Garden of Life)
- Spirulina
- Ten to twenty minutes of fresh air and exercise
- Uncorked
- Vitamin B-complex or B12

<u>Fever Relief:</u>
- Detox bath
- Cold rag on back of neck
- Peppermint and lavender essential oils on forehead and spine
- Frankincense essential oil
- Colloidal silver
- Immunity Boosters
- Wellness Tea (see recipe on page 255)
- Hydrate with coconut water

<u>Headache Remedies:</u>
- Allergy blend essential oil
- Avoid artificial fragrances and cleaners with chemicals
- Avoid refined sugars and gluten
- CBD (THC-free)
- Chiropractor
- Deep Blue essential oil
- Frankincense on thumb pad then put thumb onto roof of mouth
- Hydrate (drink half of your body weight in ounces)

- Maca root with selenium
- Magnesium
- Protein and iron should be at the right levels
- Vitamin D3

Heartburn Remedies:
- Digestive Blend essential oil
- Pinch of oatmeal on tongue (swallow)
- Raw almonds
- See Digestive Tips
- Shredded coconut in milk

Hormone Supports:
- ClaryCalm or clary sage essential oil
- Evening primrose oil
- Gaia Vitex Berry
- Gaia Women's Balance
- Holistic healing and regulation with a specialist
- Maca root with selenium
- Organic Excellence Feminine Balance Therapy

Immunity Boosters:
- Apple cider vinegar
- Bee propolis capsules or paste with Manuka honey 13+
- Bone broth
- C in high doses (10,000 IU)
- D3 (5,000 IU)
- Chopped and pressed raw garlic (take like pills)
- Dr. Oz juice or any organic green juice
- Echinacea
- Elderberry syrup
- Essential oils (On Guard, Breathe, lemon, eucalyptus)
- Extra probiotics
- Fermented foods

- Garlic (pressed and chopped)
- Greens
- Herbs and spices
- Himalayan sea salt
- Manuka honey 13+
- Mushrooms (lion's mane, chaga, reishi)
- Raw kefir
- Spices (turmeric, ginger)
- Superfood blend
- Wellness Tea (see recipe on page 255)
- Zinc

Muscle Aches, Inflammation, Joints, and Soreness Remedies:

- Arnica gel or oil
- Aroma Touch essential oil
- Castor oil packs
- CBD (THC-free)
- Chiropractor
- Coconut water (to hydrate)
- Curcumin
- Cupping
- Deep Blue essential oil
- Epsom salt bath
- Heat/ice packs and elevation
- Helichrysum essential oil
- Herbal wraps
- High doses of Turmeric Supreme Pain by Gaia
- Lemongrass
- Massage
- Red light therapy
- Stamina pro strips
- Theragun and rolling
- Vital Proteins (to help with joint health)
- Yoga and stretching

Pink Eye or Stye Remedies:

- Breastmilk in eye every two hours. If you do not have access to breastmilk, use organic raw kefir.
- Colloidal silver in eye three to six times daily
- Melaleuca and lavender on brow bone and bridge of nose
- Raw organic kefir
- Warm compress or warm tea bag compress

Sinus Infection Remedies:

- All Immunity Boosters
- Clear Products Sinus blend
- Melaleuca on Q-tip in nose as often as you can (ensure Q-tip has coconut oil on it)
- Neti Pot
- Oregano and Manuka honey 13+
- Propolis capsules
- Silver spray for the nose (use at onset of symptoms)

Skin Issues: (i.e., acne, eczema)

- Chlorella
- Get on a healing protocol
- Gold Clover tallow
- Gut healing
- Kefir (full of the best probiotics)
- Luminance skincare
- Maca root with selenium
- Metal detox

Get to the Root of the Skin Issues:

- Remove synthetics in the home
- Look into seeing if you have an omega deficiency
- Stop using traditional soaps and detergents
- Don't consume foods you're sensitive to, like gluten, corn, dairy, refined sugar, and other grains. Remember, you can

have a sensitivity or intolerance even if you don't have celiac or a full-blown allergy.

Sleep Supports:

- Bedtime tea
- Blackout shades
- Brain dump any thoughts and tasks on notepad or journal before bed
- CBD (THC-free)
- Chiropractor
- Don't drink caffeine past 2:00 PM
- Don't take a nap past 3:00 PM
- Epsom salt bath
- Get enough vitamin D and fresh air
- Get your circadian rhythm aligned
- Keep exercise to morning hours or at least not three hours before sleep
- Lavender, serenity, cedarwood, and vetiver essential oils
- Magnesium (300mg and/or transdermal spray at night)
- Make sure there are no WiFi boxes or smart meters near your room, in your room, or outside the walls of your room
- Make sure your alarm wakes you up with something calm
- Melatonin products like Sleep, Dream, Collagen shots (low doses and not long term or nightly)
- No electronics one hour before bed (put phone in airplane mode)
- Non-toxic temperature regulating sheets like Ettitude
- Ōura ring
- Red light therapy (Joovv Go)
- Routine
- Set your mind and intentions on when and how you will sleep and wake up
- Stop eating three to four hours before bed
- Stick to a sleep schedule as much as possible with the goal of six to eight hours of sleep
- Wear blue light blocking glasses
- White noise

- **Stomach Bug Remedies:**
- Activated charcoal
- Apple cider vinegar tea and black tea
- Coconut water (electrolytes)
- Colloidal silver
- Digestive Blend essential oil
- Ginger tea
- Grape seed extract (GSE)
- Lemon and peppermint essential oils (inhale)

Strep Solutions:
- Apple cider vinegar tea with grape seed extract
- Colloidal silver, take for immunity and gargle
- Elderberry
- Essential oils (On Guard topically, peppermint in tea, lavender for fever)
- Gargle with melaleuca and oregano (caution!)
- Garlic and ginger
- Goldenseal capsules: three to four capsules, four times daily
- Lemon water
- Make oregano capsules and take three times daily
- Organic raw Manuka honey 13+, one spoonful every hour
- Oregano essential oil or oregano oil capsules in high doses, never take on an empty stomach
- 1500mg pantothenic acid daily
- Propolis liquid (drop on sores)
- Propolis capsules: five to ten capsules, five to six times daily
- Rest
- Throw away chapsticks, lip glosses, and toothbrushes

Stress Relief:
- Adaptogens (ashwagandha, reishi, chaga, lion's mane)
- B vitamins
- Binaural tones

- Breathwork
- Chiropractor and massage
- CBD (THC-free)
- Detox baths with essential oils
- Digital detox
- Diet: clean eating or paleo
- Essential oils and aromatherapy
- Exercise, sun, and fresh air
- Fermented holy basil
- Herbal teas
- Maca root with selenium
- Magnesium
- Mindsets
- Mushrooms
- N-acetyl cysteine (NAC)
- Rescue Remedy
- Routine and time management
- Positive affirmations and meditations
- Sleep
- Sauna
- Self-compassion and self-care

Teething Pain Remedies:
- Baltic amber necklace
- Frozen fruits or frozen breastmilk to chew on
- Lavender essential oil and jawline
- Punkin Butt teething oil

Tooth Pain Remedies:
- Clove essential oil on tooth and gum
- Clove and salt water rinse
- CBD (THC-free)
- Lavender essential oil on jawline

Ulcer Remedies:
- Digestive Blend essential oil
- Fire Cider
- Grape seed extract (GSE)
- Specific essential oils and see Stress Relief

UTI and Bladder Infections Remedies:
- Essential oils:
  Cleansing blend topically over the urethra
  Lemongrass in water over topically over the bladder area
- Probiotics
- 100% cranberry juice or 100% blueberry juice (must be pure)
- Raw apple cider vinegar and baking soda
- Whole World Botanicals bladder support

How to Avoid UTI and Bladder Infections:
- Cotton underwear
- Daily raw apple cider vinegar
- Go to the bathroom when you need to (don't hold)
- Hydrate with water and coconut water
- Probiotics daily

Wellness Tea: (aka hot toddy, minus the vodka)
- Water (hot for tea, but you can have it cold as well)
- 1-2 Tbsp apple cider vinegar or fire cider
- 1-2 Tbsp raw honey
- 1 tsp Himalayan sea salt
- Dash of cinnamon
- Essential oils, like On Guard or oregano
- Fresh raw lemon, ginger, garlic, and turmeric

Drink as often as you want. You can even add this to green tea, other teas, or bone broth.

HOLISTIC BASICS

Appliances, Cooking, and Kitchen Essentials:
- Berkey water filter
- Blendtec or Vitamix
- Cookware (glass, cast iron, copper, stainless, and handmade, lead-free pottery ceramic), not Teflon and plastic
- Dutch oven
- French press
- Good knives
- Hand blender
- Instant Pot
- Juicer (Omega or Hurom)
- KitchenAid
- Paper towels, napkins, baking papers, bags, trash bags (recycled and compostable)
- Slow cooker
- Sponges (reusable and washable)

Kitchen and Pantry Staples:
- Aminos and enzymes
- Aloe vera juice
- Bee pollen
- Blackstrap molasses
- Bone broth
- Bragg organic apple cider vinegar
- Cacao and organic dark chocolate
- Chia seeds
- Coconut sugar
- Collagen peptides and plant proteins
- Flax seeds
- Ghee
- Grass-fed and pasture-raised meats
- Himalayan and Celtic sea salt

- Juices and smoothies
- Nitrate-free bacon
- Nut and seed butters (almond and sunflower seed)
- Pure maple syrup
- Raw grass-fed and -finished dairy (full of probiotics, omegas, and enzymes, and lactose-free)
- Raw honey and Manuka honey 13+
- Raw organic virgin cold-pressed coconut oil
- Raw organic vegetables and fruits
- Real, fermented, and cultured foods (kombucha, sauerkraut, kimchi)
- Real butter (Kerry Gold or Organic Pastures)
- Sprouted nuts, seeds, and grains
- Tahini

Go-To Cookbooks:
- *Against All Grain* by Danielle Walker
- *Celebrations* by Danielle Walker
- *Eat What You Love* by Danielle Walker
- *Keto-Paleo* by Diane Sanfilippo
- *Nom Nom Paleo* by Michelle Tam
- *Practical Paleo* by Diane Sanfilippo
- *The Autoimmune Paleo Cookbook: An Allergen-Free Approach to Managing* by Mickey Trescott
- *The 21-Day Sugar Detox: Bust Sugar & Carb Cravings Naturally* by Diane Sanfilippo
- *The Primal Kitchen* by Mark Sisson
- *The Wahls Protocol Cooking for Life* by Terry Wahls M.D.
- *The Zenbelly Cookbook* by Simone Miller
- *Thug Kitchen Cookbook* by Thug Kitchen
- *Whole Food Diary* by Kezia Neusch

CLEANING

Homemade All-Purpose Cleaner:
8oz water
4oz distilled white vinegar
15 drops melaleuca oil
15 drops lemon
Glass cleaning spray bottle

Homemade Bug Spray:
Peppermint, rosemary, and TerraShield essential oils

Homemade Glass Cleaner:
White vinegar
Distilled water
Essential oil (lemon, lime, grapefruit, wild orange, Citrus Bliss)
Glass cleaning spray bottle

Homemade Weed Killer:
Vinegar and dish soap mix

CHAPTER FIFTEEN

TESTIMONIES

JENNY

My health hit crisis-mode after I started following my doctor's orders. At the time, I had been six years free from eating sugar and flour, and drinking caffeine and alcohol. Eliminating all of that was one of the best things I did for my body.

I was also living out my dreams; I had a little girl who we spent four years doting on before I became pregnant again. All was going well with this new pregnancy until one of my appointments. My doctor strongly urged me to get the Tdap shot to protect my baby from dying of whooping cough. My doctor also recommended the flu shot. I was trying to protect my baby, so like a good mommy, I followed my doctor's suggestions.

Pretty quickly, I experienced a rash of issues—my liver enzymes spiked, blood pressure raised, I was itchy all over, blurry vision, and had streaks of red all over my skin. My body was telling me something toxic was inside of me, though I didn't know exactly why at the time. I kept contacting my doctor, but they couldn't pinpoint anything. They monitored the baby and kept sending me home.

I am embarrassed to say that at the time, I *never* thought of the vaccines. To me, I had still done the right thing to protect my baby.

Since then, I have seen the vaccine package insert that reads, "Can cause fetal harm when administered to a pregnant woman or can affect reproduction capacity." (This vaccine is now required for seventh graders to go to school. I'm pretty sure these kids will want reproduction capacity one day.) I was *not* given the package insert, nor any of the other awful possible side effects when I was strongly advised to get these shots.

At thirty-eight weeks, we lost our sweet boy after I had a placenta abruption. They said it was probably borderline HELLP syndrome and pre-eclampsia, and the doctor apologized for not listening to my pleas. We were devastated. I have since learned of an insurance whistleblower who came across death after death of babies after administering these in utero vaccines.

A year later, I became pregnant again. Healing was happening, and I was grateful I made it through with no suggested vaccinations, but the damage was already done. I had no idea how much worse it would get. My next precious boy was born, and the birth was beautiful. I was not awake though. He was vaccinated from the day he was born. He got nine vaccines bundled together (five in one, three in one, and a flu shot) at nineteen months. My boy, who was walking, talking, and eating like a champ, stopped all of those things. He stopped looking at us and talking to us. He ate only two or three things and screamed all the time. He had eczema and was falling on his head over and over, unable to maintain balance. There is more. He also got pneumonia three times before his first birthday, and received the pneumococcal vaccine three times that year. He was later diagnosed with regressive autism, but let's call it what it is—brain encephalitis. Again, we were devastated.

My daughter had also been complaining for years about body pain. We just thought it was "growing pains." Our doctor suggested we test her for Lyme disease. She had it! We couldn't believe it. We had rubbed her legs and given her ibuprofen so many times, but all along it was a disease ransacking her little body. We researched everything we could. How did she get it?

Amidst all of this, I was so tired I could barely stay awake in the day. I started to feel brain-fogged and out of it. That same doctor said to me, "Mom, you should also get tested." I was positive for Lyme disease. I have since learned that it is far more prevalent than we all know, and many people have it. It is being misdiagnosed as MS, Lupus, Fibromyalgia, and Chronic Fatigue Syndrome. The CDC standards for testing are a rabbit hole I never wanted to go down. But having done it, I know why we have Lyme and why people go years chasing a diagnosis, yet don't find the proper one. It is life-changing, and most people have no idea the devastation Lyme disease brings.

Why all the sickness in my little family? We all went through genetic testing after our diagnoses. We have the MTHFR gene mutation, and I have the most severe form. We do not methylate properly, and therefore do not detox well. We weren't able to rid our bodies of the toxins in vaccines: the aluminum, formaldehyde, polysorbate 80, and mercury (thimerosal) in the flu shots. I can't even think about the aborted fetal cells, which means foreign DNA in our bodies, bovine serum, MSG, and monkey kidney cells.

Since our diagnoses, we have found amazing people who know how to detox the body, supply it with what it needs to function optimally, and we have been on the road to recovery. It is a full-time job to be healthy for us. It means infrared sauna, essential oils, and Ion Cleanse footbaths for detoxing heavy metals, pesticides, mold, and candida. It means chiropractic care, cranial work, and working with naturopathic doctors. It means lining our home with non-toxic everything, including food. Organic and non-GMO foods are a must to be free from ingesting pesticides. It's not cheap, but it's worth the investment.

Within two weeks of going organic, gluten-free, and dairy-free, my four-year-old son started speaking in full sentences, after using gibberish to communicate prior. It was amazing progress and incredibly eye-opening! It felt like a whirlwind going toxin-free, but once we did it, we were on a roll. We are never going back.

I learned the hard way to ask questions, to trust my instincts, and to have confidence in my decisions. I trusted those who went before me, and those who knew about clean living well before I did. Most of us learned the hard way, but I'm not alone in my endeavor to protect my family.

KARA

In 2013, I went to my doctor with severe abdominal pain. I was twenty-three years old and weighed 338 pounds. After several tests, my doctor concluded that I had a fatty liver and suggested I get gastric bypass surgery. I was terrified and refused the surgery. I had it in my head that if I ate my way into this, I would eat my way out!

After one year of calorie counting and going to the gym three to five days a week, I lost 60 pounds but still had abdominal pain. I went back to my doctor to talk about the increasing pain and received a second diagnosis. This time it was not my liver, but my gallbladder—the original and missed source to the pain I walked in with one year prior.

My gallbladder was extremely low in function, and both my doctor and a surgeon advised me that it would be best to get the gallbladder removed. I asked about natural routes and was told there were none. Because I was an advocate for my own body and ended up refusing the surgery to explore natural options, I was called an *experiment*.

The same week of my second diagnosis, Chrissy hosted her 2014 Flourish Health Summit, and I decided I would attend. I went to one of the breakout sessions on gut health. The speaker, Christine Andrews, was a holistic nutritionist who worked in town. I pulled her aside at the end and explained my condition to her in hopes that she would have answers, and she did!

I met with Christine one-on-one for several months. She helped me get aggressive with losing weight, and gave me natural supplements to target and heal my gallbladder and liver. After feeling such a significant difference in my health, I went back to my doctor and repeated the same tests I took in 2013. To her amazement, my gallbladder had doubled in function! Shocked and answerless, I was sent to a surgeon for a second opinion, and because of his amazement, he voted I keep the gallbladder in and stick to the holistic side.

Post Flourish, I received the privilege of working alongside Chrissy for two years at her holistic boutique, Eco Chic. I learned and gleaned holistic health wisdom from her and the Eco Chic team! I was saturated in a positive, like-minded, and passionate health environment. There, I not only completed a physical healing and realignment but a spiritual one! These two things were connected and at the root of the disease that tried to take my life prematurely.

Since I began my journey, I've lost a total of 160 pounds naturally and slowly, my gallbladder is restored, and my liver is doing great! I decided to continue to channel my passion and drive for health and return to school to study nutrition at Sacramento State University. Without Chrissy and the connections I have made through her, I would not be where I am at today. I am completely honored to have walked out this journey and truly believe it was all a gift from above!

DAVID

As a young adult, I'm implementing clean eating, natural wellness, and consistent exercise into my life now to take a proactive approach to my overall health. It's my duty to be a good steward of my mind, body, and spirit. I find that eating clean, supplementing with natural herbs and vitamins, exercising, and taking care of my mind is helping reduce my stress levels and increasing my productivity throughout the day.

REBECCA

Getting to where I am now was very much a process. Four months after I had my first baby, I started experiencing intense lower back pain. I went to the ER because I almost couldn't walk. They took one look at me and told me it was because I was fat, and that was it. I walked out of the ER embarrassed, ashamed, hurt, and unheard. That propelled me to become an expert on my health.

I started looking at household products first, and realized I needed to change my environment. I was horrified to see what companies were putting not only in products adults use, but what they were promoting we use on our babies and children! My mama bear came out like none other! I started swapping out products as fast as I could. That led me to investigate food and what I was consuming and feeding my family.

I learned what to look out for and read a lot of books. I changed my way of life, from purchasing safer products to implementing healthier foods and exercising regularly. I was also developing myself consistently and growing spiritually.

In February 2016, God called our family to move from Kansas City to Northern California because He had our purpose out here! Over a year and a half, I lost 110 pounds and felt better than ever, but I *still* had random lower back pain that wouldn't go away no matter what I did. I had debilitating, life-stopping flare-ups once every few months.

In 2017, I assumed I'd always have this mysterious pain, and this was my lot in life. That July, I found out I was expecting baby number two, and the same week I found out, I had another one of those horrendous flare-ups. Going into my pregnancy, I was ignorant of what was about to take place. I was at a healthy weight, exercising regularly, and eating well. I was convinced I was going to have an amazing and easy pregnancy, and I was going to bounce back right after the baby was delivered. I assumed my labor and delivery experience was going to be a piece of cake! Poor, ignorant self; I have so much compassion and grace for that mama.

My pregnancy was full of non-stop pain and extreme fatigue that never subsided, even in the wonder months (months four through seven). I couldn't sleep at night and couldn't sleep enough during the day. All I wanted to do was eat junk food. I couldn't exercise anymore because my hips were in constant pain, and I couldn't even clean my house without hurting for three days.

The birthing process for this baby was a major trauma; I had PTSD from that experience. I also had to make the very difficult decision I couldn't have kids anymore because my body was totaled.

I wanted freedom from the sugar addition I'd gained from pregnancy, so I started researching holistic practices for eating and living. I found a paleo and keto sugar detox approach, and pledged to myself that I'd do that for six months—and I did!

Through those six months, I learned exponentially more about holistic health than I could have imagined! I learned that I have an autoimmune disease and removing gluten, conventional dairy, sugar of any kind, hydrogenated oils, corn, and birth control has saved my body from those painful flare-ups. Having answers is the most liberating thing. I've found my calling and purpose, and now I'm well enough and healed enough to live out that God-given purpose!

Because of the PTSD from my birthing experience, I developed postpartum anxiety, which left me in fear of leaving my house. All I could do was imagine all the things that could go wrong if I left my home, especially with my boys. I started listening to holistic wellness podcasts daily, multiple times a day, in fact.

I was healing, and I got the courage to apply to work for Chrissy at Eco Chic so I could start helping other people live their best lives as well! I can't even believe how different things are now from where I was a year ago. I'm so grateful for what holistic health has done for my family and me, and I love that I get to share that information with others!

CHRISTINA

Looking back on my health journey, the craziest part was how disconnected I was from my body. I couldn't tell you when my last menstrual cycle was, or if it came at all. I couldn't tell how certain foods made me feel, or what my body was trying to tell me if I felt something "off." I didn't spend much time trying to get to know my body's voice, or investing in taking care of it. That was until my body spoke so loud I had to listen, "Christina, we have cancer." I felt heartbroken, betrayed, and blindsided. Had there been warning signs? Had my body been trying to speak to me years prior, and was I too busy to listen? I have thought about that often, and I still don't know. What I did know was that I heard it loud and clear, and this time I needed to make a change.

I'm an all-or-nothing kind of gal. So, when I decided I was going to start giving my body the nourishment and attention it deserved, I dove in head first, reading every book I could find on the topic of wellness and holistic health. I wasn't looking for love, but I found it there. I was enamored by the body's desire and ability to heal when given the opportunity to do so, and at the same time, I was infuriated by the corruption and neglect of the pharmaceutical companies and major food suppliers. I had been blind to the slow and silent poisoning of my Diet Coke addiction and pesticide- and GMO-ridden "healthy vegetarian diet" for the previous decade. That was the end of it for me. The curtain was torn back, and I felt empowered and awake. I decided to live the rest of my days honoring my body, the earth, and future generations with the food I ate, and I was committed to educate and empower anyone who would listen.

It's been almost eight years since I began my healing journey, and it's one I will continue for the rest of my life. Health requires showing up for yourself every day. It's not a destination you reach, but a lifestyle you walk out in the food you eat, relationships you have, boundaries you set, and all the ways you tend to your body's ever-changing needs. It's not always fast and easy, but it's so worth it. Life done intentionally is a life well-lived. What's your intention? Is it to feel good, look better, have more peace, get off your medications, apologize more, work through your grief, or start exercising? Whatever it is, start today! Start right now! Your body will thank you.

ASHLEY

Western medicine completely failed me. After suffering postpartum anxiety and severe fatigue, no doctor was truly able to provide any assistance; they only wanted to throw medication at me to band-aid my symptoms. That wasn't good enough for me. Not only am I a minimalist when it comes to medications, but I wanted a long-term solution. Because of this, I took my wellness into my own hands to search for real solutions.

Through trial and error, and the support of my sisterhood around me, I finally found complete relief of my fatigue, anxiety, and gut issues. I started on a whole foods and balanced diet, proper supplements, lifestyle changes (like meditation, yoga, and acupuncture), and increased my physical activity. I'm so grateful I knew myself enough to know that there was a better solution than suppressing my symptoms with medications. I healed myself from the inside out.

LINDSI

I was most intentional with my health journey after I had my first baby. I've always had a grid for what being healthy was, but it intensified when I became a mother. Here was this new life; a tiny, fragile person who relied on me for life and safety.

The first things to change were my cleaning products. I didn't want her to breathe in poison or crawl on a floor cleaned with harsh chemicals. And when she was ready for solid food, I made it myself, because that's what my mom did for me.

After her birth, I was suddenly confronted with exhaustion and postpartum depression. I felt like I was barely making it through each day, but I didn't know how to fix it. I struggled to keep up with exercise, and I felt lost in my postpartum body, completely overwhelmed with motherhood.

Besides the fact I took prenatal vitamins and tried to eat healthy during pregnancy, vitamins were not something I normally took. Within that first year, my dad started me on some natural supplements that completely turned my life around. My brain fog cleared and my energy came back. I started enjoying life again. This was the first stepping stone on a journey to constantly learning and adding to my health.

I took small steps in making changes without any internet research; I just followed my gut. It's like a lightbulb turned on and I could see how the environment could affect my baby. She was so pure, and why would I put anything in her that could mess with that?

As time went on, I wanted to have another baby, but I was locked in fear of having another C-section, so I waited. I went through a season of battling with this fear, yet wanting another baby. *Could there be another way? Did I have to have a C-section again?*

I asked Chrissy what exactly she did in regard to birth. She explained she was a doula, and pretty much from that moment forward, I had a peace wash over me, letting me know I could have a safe home birth.

My study and pursuit of home birth is where my health journey accelerated. I met my midwife, and she opened my eyes to a world of healthy alternatives for moms and babies. I read *Ina May's Guide to Childbirth* and realized birth is so much more than "getting the baby out." It's about a healthy mom and baby. It's about women supporting women, and families thriving. It's about allowing the body to do what it was made to do. So what does this have to do with a healthy lifestyle? Everything.

With each baby, I learned something new about health because

I wanted the best for my kids and the best for myself as a mother. I wanted successful births, and natural products on hand so I could handle things like mastitis, diaper rash, milk supply issues, fever, and postpartum healing without rushing to a doctor's office.

I sought chiropractic care, and recommend it to all expecting moms. Joint pain is real in pregnancy, but it doesn't have to be. Pregnancy is not a medical condition that needs fixing. It is a natural, beautiful time that brings life into the world. Of course, there are times when moms and babies need medical attention and emergency C-sections. I'm not downplaying that at all. I am saying that in many cases, moms are fearful when they are doing great and their baby is healthy, but the hospital system can create fear around due dates, gestational diabetes, breech babies, pain during labor, and a lot of *what-ifs*. Home birth taught me to enjoy pregnancy and to trust my body, find alternatives to conventional medications, and to nourish my body with good fats and organic foods.

I learn something new about health every day. One thing I will always stick to is listening to my body (not following fad diets but looking at food as medicine). Also, I've learned to not do the same workout as Suzy, who might look healthy, but she's really just stressing her body out more and getting even sicker. Another thing I stick to is resting when I need to, and applying my routine of self-care.

Chiropractic care will always be part of my life. My immune system functions best when my nervous system is in alignment. I went through a frustrating season of catching frequent colds, even though I was doing all the right things. My chiropractor says, "Health is not about how we *feel*, but about how we *heal*."

We discovered the area of my spine that supports my immune system was stressed and not communicating with my brain, so my brain didn't know what to do to fight infection! My body was made to heal, and after consistent chiropractic care and some exercises at home, my immune system is back to functioning the way God made it to! Now my supplements are more effective, and my body recognizes healing foods better!

KIMBERLIE

I was raised on meals that mostly came from boxes and cans. I grew up having painful eczema, silent GERD (gastroesophageal reflux disease), chronic bronchitis, and embarrassing digestive issues. I didn't learn I had GERD until I got married and started a family. That time was also when I began to hear about alternative medicine.

My firstborn projectile vomited whenever I ate dairy, and had reflux and colic for over a year. In my last trimester with another one of my children, I woke up every night choking and gasping for air, nearly blacking out. Doctors thought it was asthma until I finally talked to a GI specialist who told me about GERD and described my exact symptoms.

I was so emotional thinking about all the years of suffering. This new knowledge sent me deep into research on processed foods, genetics, and chemicals from our environment and household products we used daily. I was amazed at how cutting out gluten and processed dairy could help my body heal from eczema and GERD.

When my children were toddlers, I slowly learned about the toxic ingredients found in most vaccines. I was heartbroken that I was never informed in the doctor's office; I just took their word that it was safe. I found out my children were vaccine injured because of their colic, asthma, chronic ear infections, and uncontrollable crying for the first years of their lives. Weeks after their injections they had behavioral changes and uncontrollable shaking and screaming.

We were recently tested, due to our genetics, and we discovered we have gene mutations and food allergies that look different than others. Due to the ingredients in vaccines, we learned it's not just harmful, but life-threatening for us to receive them.

I'm grateful to now know the truth. We have to take our health into our own hands and not rely on others. Don't be afraid to ask questions, do your research, get tested, and be intentional to advocate for yourself and your children.

CHAPTER SIXTEEN

HEALTH AFFIRMATIONS

I am at peace, and I bring peace wherever I go.
I am worthy.
I will dream big and never settle.
I was born to make an impact.
I wake up with energy, hope, clarity, and joy.
I carry greatness and miracles inside of me.
I am loved.
I am thankful for my health journey and the resources available to me.
I will accept more and judge less.
I have peace, love, power, and a sound mind.
I am blessed.
I was made to do hard and brave things.
I am doing a great job.
I am loved and appreciated.
I am enough.
I am not alone.
I will be kind to everyone I encounter.
I have an abundance of hope and joy in my life.

I will make time for what makes me come alive.

I am capable.

I can do hard things.

I have the abundance and resources needed to take care of myself.

I have the power to change, heal, and be whole.

I feel stronger and healthier every day.

I make wise and healthy choices daily.

I love myself, and I am perfectly healthy.

My mind, body, and spirit are in total alignment.

I forgive and release those who have offended, wounded, left, or hurt me in some way.

I am vigorous and full of energy, clarity, and focus.

I am radically healthy and radiant.

I operate at a high level of success, peace, and favor.

I am a grateful and thankful person.

I am the nicest, kindest, and most positive person in each room every day.

I am awakened to truth and will make decisions that benefit my body, mind, spirit, home, and future.

I am a co-creator and leader.

I think, speak, act, and live from health and abundance.

I am strong, I am able, and I am powerful to choose well.

I consume things that are healthy, nourishing, and healing to my body.

I protect my peace, my energy, and my heart.

I make health a priority every day.

I give myself permission to heal and walk in wholeness.

I am worthy of better choices, better thoughts, a better body, and a better life.

I release all disappointment, shame, guilt, anger, bitterness, resentment, and limiting beliefs.

I am slow to anger, slow to judge, and slow to offend.

I am quick to forgive.

I am quick to heal.

I have a strong immune system, my hormones are in alignment, and my gut is healed.

I crave truth, healthy foods, healthy people, and peace.

I am not defined by my mistakes.

I am humble, kind, peaceful, and compassionate.

I release all expectations and attachments.

I will make my dreams actionable, and I will make my voice heard.

I am patient with myself and the process.

I choose to trust in my journey.

I am brilliant, resilient, wise, and determined.

I breathe in peace, wisdom, and love. I exhale confusion, stress, and pain.

I am making a difference with good decisions every day.

I am healthy, healed, and whole.

My mind, body, spirit, and emotions are healing, transforming, and elevating for my highest good.

I do what is right, not what is easy.

I respond with empathy, compassion, grace, and understanding.

I am in charge of me. I get to choose how I feel. I am powerful.

CHAPTER SEVENTEEN

CHALLENGE AND COMMISSION

"Think different."
— *Steve Jobs*

This book is not just a book. It's a call; it's a charge. It's been said that a book is a conversation with the author, and I pray you have enjoyed our talk. We got really close, real fast, didn't we? There are things you probably didn't agree with or you're not sure about, and that's great because now you can do more research and make your own powerful decisions.

This isn't a book you read; this is a book you live. A book you give. A book you reference back to. This isn't a book you skimmed through and laughed through—okay some parts you laughed through (at least I hope). You picked up this book because it called you, or because you're my friend. That's cool, too, and I thank you *deeply*. This book isn't meant to be read once and shelved away. I wrote it to be revisited, tweeted, repeated, ran with, prayed over, and shared. It's meant to be applied, not just applauded. (Please do applaud, though. Especially on Amazon, so it sells y'all!) It's meant to be highlighted and written in.

Its purpose is to bring light, wisdom, honor, truth, strategy, and success to your heart, mind, spirit, and body.

If you thought this was a book just about "organic," you found it wasn't, and I'm glad you stayed with it through the end. Thank you. The power is now in your hands and your heart. What will you do with this depth of insight, inspiration, and information? What will you do with your new level of awareness? What will you do with your new wisdom?

I dare you to:
Share.
Do.
Act.
Live.
Go.

ACKNOWLEDGMENTS

With any "baby," there is always a birth team. This is my first real "book baby," and I would not have been able to complete this book at the level it's at without very key people in my corner and on my team. Writing this book was an incredible process, and I'm excited about the future books to come.

In all honesty, the time of writing this book was a pretty hard season in my personal life and business. Thankfully, I didn't let that stop me from pouring my all into this book. The journey was incredible as I was able to apply and be reminded of every tool and tip as I was in the thick of it. Living out and implementing the insights in this book *works*. I know firsthand, as so much of me was tested beyond the usual in this process. I don't think you can write a book without having battles, growth, and upgrades—at least that was my experience. I realize this is the longest acknowledgment in the history of book acknowledgments, but remember gratitude and honor are everything.

It's always God above everything for me. So thank you, Jesus.

Literally, I likely would not even be on this planet or a healthy, amazing human without the grace, truth, love, and power of God in every detail of my life.

To you, the reader, thank you. Thank you for living these words and supporting this mission to see wholeness in every heart and home.

I give my deepest thank you to Josh, Gabe, Noah, Mercy, and Zoe. You guys are my greatest teachers, inspiration, and motivation. You put up with my crazy like no other. You all bring something valuable, special, and irreplaceable to my journey and life. I love you more than you will ever know.

Thank you to my parents for raising a leader and never shutting me down. You have always been my biggest fans and supporters. I am grateful for you. I also forgive you for the Lucky Charms. You are incredible people, amazing grandparents, and friends. I love you so much. Thank you to all my extended family, including the best sister and mother-in-law a girl could ever have.

Thank you to my uncle who showed me how to dream radically big, love bigger, and give generously. He always supported my crazy, my passions, and my voice growing up. It truly shaped who I am. I know he would be proud. He would have bought nine million copies of this book. I know it.

Thank you to my Eco Chic team who have been incredibly supportive and encouraging during the writing of this book, and in every high and low we have had together this last year. I would not have been able to write this book at this level without your prayers, love, and help.

Thank you to my BFFFFFFF—you are my soul sister. I love you. Thank you to my tribe. You know who you are. You have championed me, prayed for me, sent me words on just the right day, kicked my butt, held me accountable, gave me valuable feedback, pushed me, loved me, showed up for me, and encouraged me like no other. I love you so much—to infinity and beyond with you gems.

Thank you to my pastors from childhood to today who spoke so much life and truth into me. You saw something in me even when I tried to run from it as a teenager. Your words have helped heal, shape, and awaken things inside of me. Thank you for your prayers, support, encouragement, and wisdom. Thank you to my mentor and therapist who has truly helped me transform my inner world and life.

Thank you to my customers and clients who have been on a ten-year-plus journey with me. You have been loyal, faithful, supportive, and consistent; I have so much love for you.

Thank you to the world's best editor. This book wouldn't even be close to what it is without your wisdom, gifts, time, and heart. Let's write a hundred more. You are the best.

Thank you to the many mentors I have had: online, masterminds, life coaches, inner circles, groups, round tables, small groups, and beyond. It has all added value to my life, business, and this book. Many greats have deeply inspired me, and their influence is weaved through these pages as well.

Thank you to my failures, haters, betrayers, dead dreams, mistakes, misguided passions, broken relationships, and horrible days. You brought me here. I never lost, but I sure learned a lot.

I also want to acknowledge and thank myself for sticking with my goal, executing, pressing through, overcoming, rising above, living every word in this book, being in the 5 AM Club, not shrinking back, and not backing down, no matter the resistance. I am proud of you.

GLOSSARY

BDNF: Brain-derived neurotrophic factor

Big Pharma: Pharmaceutical companies collectively, as a sector of the industry

Broken brain: Coined by Dr. Mark Hyman, the manifestation of depression, anxiety, ADHD, ADD, autism, Alzheimer's, bipolar, and many other mental disorders that could be prevented with functional medicine and diet

Detox: Abstaining from or ridding the body of toxic or un-healthy substances

Doula: A certified birth coach

EEG: (electroencephalography) An electrophysiological moni-toring method to record electrical activity of the brain

EMF/Radiation: Electromagnetic field, electronic waves

Gene mutation: Alteration of genes in the DNA sequence, dif-ferent than most people. These cause health issues or trouble processing certain things.

Geoengineering/chemtrails: Visible trail left in the sky full of chemicals and biological agents that can cause health issues, and disrupt weather, or create weather patterns. Normal clouds do not make zigzags or lines.

GI: Gastrointestinal collective of the stomach, small intestine, and large intestine.

Greenwash: Disinformation disseminated by an organization that presents itself as ethical, organic, or environmentally responsible for image purposes

IUD: Intrauterine device used for birth control

Fibroids: Benign tumors made up of connective tissue

LED: Light-emitting diode, a type of artificial light

Mold: Fungus that grows and releases spores

Neurogenesis: Generation of cells, a growth, and development of nervous tissue

RSV: Respiratory Syncytial Virus

SAD diet: Standard American Diet

Woke: Alert to injustice, waking up from a state of sleep, become aware of, causing something to stir, or come to life

WIC: Women, Infants, and Children food stamps

RESOURCES

INTRODUCTION
Books:
The Road Back to You by Ian Morgan Cron and Suzanne Stabile
The Sacred Enneagram by Christopher L. Heuertz

Websites:
Enneagram test   https://www.yourenneagramcoach.com/

CHAPTER ONE
Books:
Patient Heal Thyself by Dr. Jordan Rubin
Start With Why by Simon Sinek

Documentaries:
Heal
Stink!
The Greater Good
The Truth About Cancer
Trace Amounts
Vaxxed: From Cover-Up to Catastrophe

Websites:
Dr. Ben Lynch   https://www.drbenlynch.com
Weston A. Price Foundation   https://www.westonaprice.org

CHAPTER TWO
Books:
The 5 AM Club by Robin Sharma

Local Farms:
Be Love Farm   http://belovefarm.com
Casa Rosa Farm   http://www.casarosafarm.net
Eatwell Farm   http://www.eatwell.com
Lockewood Acres   7781 Locke Rd, Vacaville, CA 95688

Websites:
Kristin Neff, Self-Compassion   https://self-compassion.org
Gayle Belanger, Live Free   https://www.livefreeministry.org
Non-LED light bulbs   https://www.acehardware.com

CHAPTER THREE
Websites:
Andrea Thompson   https://andreathompson.org
Dann Farrelly   http://bit.ly/DannFarrelly
Danny Silk   https://www.lovingonpurpose.com
Gottman   https://www.gottman.com/

CHAPTER FOUR
Books:
Feeding You Lies by Vani Hari
Ina May's Guide to Childbirth by Ina May Gaskin
Kiss the Ground by Josh Tickell

Websites:
Birth Control   http://bit.ly/syntheticbirthcontrol
Environmental Working Group (EWG)   https://ewg.org
Food Babe Blog   https://foodbabe.com
Vaccines   http://bit.ly/BillGatesVaccine

Documentaries:
Broken Brain
Business of Being Born
Fed Up

Food Inc.
Unplanned
Why Not Home?

Services:
New Life Birth Services   http://www.newlifebirthservices.org
Austin Doula Collective   http://www.austindoulacollective.com

CHAPTER FIVE

Books:
Conscious Language by Robert Tennyson Stevens
Radiation Nation by Daniel T Debaun and Ryan P. Debaun

Podcasts:
Broken Brain, Dr. Mark Hyman, Episode #39
Healing From Mold Exposure, Medical Medium

Documentaries:
An Inconvenient Tooth
Fluoridegate: An American Tragedy
Root Cause

Websites:
Bio Balance Now   http://biobalancenow.com
Breast Cancer Action   https://bcaction.org
Botox   http://bit.ly/whynotbotox
CritiSafe   www.citrisafe.com
Dr. Ann Shippy   https://annshippymd.com/mold/
GENIE test   http://bit.ly/GENIEtest
Hair Salons   http://bit.ly/hairdyes
Hormones   http://bit.ly/nickelallergy
Mammograms   http://bit.ly/mammogramdanger
MTHFR Pregnancy   http://bit.ly/MTHFRpregnancy
Susan Komen   http://bit.ly/SusanKomenOncology

Vaccines   http://www.vactruth.com/
Vaccines   www.LearnTheRisk.org/diseases

<u>**Services:**</u>
Northern California EMF Professional http://bit.ly/EMFprofessional

CHAPTER SIX

<u>**Books:**</u>
Digital Minimalism by Cal Newport
Poverty, Riches and Wealth by Kris Vallotton
Screen Schooled by Joe Clement and Matt Miles

<u>**Podcasts:**</u>

Hack to Track: The Ōura Ring Episode, Bulletproof Radio, Episode #536
How Social Media May Be Ruining Your Life, The Doctor's Farmacy, Episode #39

<u>**Apps:**</u>
EveryDollar
Mint: Personal Finance & Money
YNAB (You Need A Budget)

<u>**Documentaries:**</u>
Minimalism: A Documentary About the Important Things
Screenagers
Tidying Up with Marie Kondo

<u>**Websites:**</u>
Collin Kartchner TED Talk   http://bit.ly/collinTEDtalk
Diet Fitness Pro   https://www.dnafit.com/us/store/dietfitnesspro.asp
DNAFit   https://www.dnafit.com/us/
#SavetheKids   https://savethekids.us
Simon Sinek TED Talk   http://bit.ly/sinekTEDtalk
Smartphone Addiction   http://bit.ly/breaksmartphoneaddiction

Services:
Maximum Fitness   https://www.maximumfitnessvacaville.com

CHAPTER SEVEN
Podcasts:
Dr. Zach Bush M.D. — Gut Health and the Microbiome, Collective Insights, Episode #17

CHAPTER EIGHT
Books:
Digging the Wells of Revival by Lou Engle
Immortal Diamond by Richard Rohr
Possessing the Gates of the Enemy by Cindy Jacobs
Rees Howells: Intercessor by Norman Grubb
Switch On Your Brain by Dr. Caroline Leaf
The Practice of the Presence of God by Brother Lawrence
Watchman Prayer by Dutch Sheets
What the Mystics Know by Richard Rohr

Apps:
BrainWave: 35 Binaural Series™
Calm
Headspace: Meditation & Sleep
Soultime Christian Meditation

Podcasts:
Kwik Brain, Jim Kwik

CHAPTER NINE
Books:
Self-Compassion by Kristin Neff
Practice You: A Journal by Elena Brower

CHAPTER THIRTEEN

Books:

Brain Body Diet by Sara Gottfried

Podcasts:

Born to Impact, Joel Marion
Broken Brain, Dr. Mark Hyman and Dhru Purohit
Bulletproof Radio, Dave Asprey
Collective Insights, Neurohacker
Ed Mylett Show
Elevation Church, Steven Furtick
Fun Therapy, Mike Foster
Go Beyond
Impact Theory, Tom Bilyeu
Jon Gordon
Kevin Rose
Kwik Brain
Loving on Purpose
Mindvalley
Model Health Show
Mosaic, Erwin McManus
Next Level Living, Chrissy Helmer
Super Soul Sunday, Oprah Winfrey
Take Control of Your Health, Dr. Joseph Mercola
The Brian Buffini Show
The Doctor's Farmacy, Dr. Mark Hyman
The Dr. Gundry Podcast
The Microbiome Reports
The Playbook with David Meltzer
The Vaccine Conversation, Melissa and Dr. Bob
Win Today, Christopher Cook

REFERENCES

CHAPTER ONE

"According to Dr. John Bergman" — Spencer, Stephan. "Avoiding and Reversing Disease Through Alternative Health Therapies with John Bergman." Get Yourself Optimized, 7 Jan. 2016, www.getyourselfoptimized.com/avoiding-and-reversing-disease-through-alternative-health-therapies-john-bergman/.

"This is because, for many people's bodies," — Real Food Forager. "6 Reasons to NEVER Eat Corn Especially for Celiac." Real Food Forager, 24 Jan. 2018, realfoodforager.com/6-reasons-to-never-eat-corn-especially-if-you-are-celiac-or-gluten-sensitive-2/.

CHAPTER TWO

"First sixty minutes of your day" — Sharma, Robin S. The 5 AM Club: Own Your Morning, Elevate Your Life. HarperCollinsPublishers, 2018.

CHAPTER THREE

"adjective warmly or deeply appreciative" — "Grateful." Dictionary.com, Dictionary.com, www.dictionary.com/browse/grateful.

"I believe those with healthy" — Sharma, Robin S. The 5 AM Club: Own Your Morning, Elevate Your Life. HarperCollinsPublishers, 2018.

"Benefits of being positive" — Gordon, Jon. "The Benefits of Positivity and Cost of Negativity." Jon Gordon: The Positive Dog, 2 June 2014, jongordon.com/positive-tip-benefits-cost.html.

"Up to 90 percent of illness" — Leaf, Caroline. "You Are What You Think." Dr. Caroline Leaf, 30 Nov. 2011, drleaf.com/blog/single-entry/print/you-are-what-you-think-75-98-of-mental-and-physical-illnesses-come-from-our-thought-life/.

CHAPTER FOUR

"Officials from the FDA" — Linklater, Richard, director. Fast Food Nation. World Cinema Ltd, 2007.

"We hardwire our brain to crave sugar" — Schaefer, Anna, and Kareem Yasin. "Is Sugar the Next 'Street Drug'?" Healthline, Healthline Media, 10 Oct. 2016, www.healthline.com/health/food-nutrition/experts-is-sugar-addictive-drug.

"As Jason Vale says in *Hungry For Change*" — Vale, Jason. "Sugar Is a Drug." Hungry For Change, 2013, www.hungryforchange.tv/article/sugar-is-a-drug.

"...whatever goes into the sewer system" — Orlando, Laura. "It's Time to Talk (Again) about Sewage Sludge on Farmland." In These Times, 11 July 2017, inthesetimes.com/rural-america/entry/20319/sewage-sludge-biosolids-public-health-waste-management-agriculture.

"Like I mentioned, fetal parts" — Harkness, Kelsey. "In the Market for Fetal Body Parts, a Baby's Brain Sells for $3,340." LifeNews.com, 20 Apr. 2016, www.lifenews.com/2016/04/20/in-the-market-for-fetal-body-parts-a-babys-brain-sells-for-3340/.

"For starters, Americans pay more for their healthcare" — Kliff, Sarah. "8 Facts That Explain What's Wrong With American Health Care."

Schwartzreport, 8 Sept. 2014, www.schwartzreport.net/8-facts-that-explain-whats-wrong-with-american-health-care/.

"In 1999, the Institute of Medicine" — Palatnik, AnneMarie. "To Err IS Human : Nursing2019 Critical Care." LWW, Oxford University Press, Sept. 2016, journals.lww.com/nursingcriticalcare/Fulltext/2016/09000/To_err_IS_human.1.aspx.

"A follow-up study published" — Allen, Marshall. "How Many Die From Medical Mistakes In U.S. Hospitals?" NPR, NPR, 20 Sept. 2013, www.npr.org/blogs/health/2013/09/20/224507654/how-many-die-from-medical-mistakes-in-u-s-hospitals.

"Did you know 90 percent" — Buttorff C, Ruder T, Bauman M. Multiple Chronic Conditions in the United States. External. Santa Monica, CA: Rand Corp., 2017.; Center for Medicare & Medicaid Services. National Health Expenditure Data for 2016—Highlights.

"Integrative medicine shifts the emphasis" — Sutter Health. "Activate the Healing Potential Ofyour Body, Mind and Spirit." CPMC Kidney Disease and Nephrology | Sutter Health, 2018, www.sutterhealth.org/lp/ihh/.

"There are tens of thousands of unsafe chemicals" — "The Never List™." Beautycounter, 2019, www.beautycounter.com/the-never-list.

"I'm not exaggerating when I say" — Mercola, Dr. Joseph. "Perfumed Poison: the Hidden Dangers of Fragrances." Dr. Joseph Mercola on Natural Health Products and Articles, 13 Feb. 2012, www.drmercola.com/health-tips/perfumed-poison-the-hidden-dangers-of-fragrances/.

"When we repeatedly expose our bodies" — "Are Tampons Toxic?" Goop, 1 Nov. 2018, goop.com/wellness/sexual-health/are-tampons-toxic/.

"The lowest year for births" — Chappell, Bill. "U.S. Births Dip To 30-Year Low; Fertility Rate Sinks Further Below Replacement Level." NPR, NPR, 17 May 2018, www.npr.org/sections/thetwo-way/2018/05/17/611898421/u-s-births-falls-to-30-year-low-sending-fertility-rate-to-a-record-low.

"Abortion is the leading cause" — Rose, Lila. "The Leading Cause of Death Globally in 2018 Wasn't Cancer, Heart Disease, HIV/AIDs or Traffic Accidents. It Was Abortion. Over 41 Million Children Killed before Birth." Twitter, Twitter, 14 Jan. 2019, twitter.com/LilaGrace-Rose/status/1084605484181716992.

Photos — "Regenerative Farming." Kiss the Ground, 2018, kiss-theground.com/regeneration/.

"Over seventy thousand people died" — "New Data Show Growing Complexity of Drug Overdose Deaths in America | CDC Online Newsroom | CDC." Centers for Disease Control and Prevention, Centers for Disease Control and Prevention, 21 Dec. 2018, www.cdc.gov/media/releases/2018/p1221-complexity-drug-overdose.html.

CHAPTER FIVE

"To give you a taste of how important" — Aggarwal. Cancer Is a Preventable Disease That Requires Major Lifestyle Changes, Sept. 2008, www.ncbi.nlm.nih.gov/pmc/articles/PMC2515569/.

"There are seventeen million new cases" — "Worldwide Cancer Statistics." Stages | Mesothelioma | Cancer Research UK, 14 Nov. 2018, www.cancerresearchuk.org/health-professional/cancer-statistics/worldwide-cancer.

"It has a long history of being an enemy" — Asprey, Dave. "My Flood Story and What to Do About Mold." Bulletproof, Bulletproof, 9 Nov.

2017, blog.bulletproof.com/my-flood-story-and-what-to-do-about-mold/.

"Symptoms of Toxic Mold" — Asprey, Dave. Moldy. Moldy, 2015, moldymovie.com.

"Avoid These Mold-Prone Foods" — William, Anthony. Medical Medium: Secrets Behind Chronic and Mystery Illness and How to Finally Heal. Hay House Inc, 2017.

"Studies show that the polycyclic" — "Black Tattoos Entail Substantial Uptake of Genotoxicpolycyclic Aromatic Hydrocarbons (PAH) in Human Skin and Regional Lymph Nodes." Edited by Fernando Rodrigues-Lima, NCIB, 26 Mar. 2014, www.ncbi.nlm.nih.gov/pmc/articles/PMC3966813/.

"Excess copper can create symptoms" — "Copper Deficiency or Toxicity..." Copper Toxicity, 2019, coppertoxic.com/symptoms.

"The reality is that mammograms only save" — Mercola, Joseph. "Mammography False Alarms Linked with Later Tumor Risk." Mercola.com, Mercola.com, 16 Sept. 2014, articles.mercola.com/sites/articles/archive/2014/09/16/mammogram-false-positive-rate.aspx.

"LED lighting may be one of the most critical" — Mercola, Joseph. "You Likely Use These Eye-Destroying Light Bulbs Not Realizing They're Linked to Blindness." Mercola.com, Mercola.com, 23 Oct. 2016, articles.mercola.com/sites/articles/archive/2016/10/23/near-infrared-led-lighting.aspx.

"World Health Organization now classifies" — Zerbe, Leah. "What Are Cell Phones Doing to Our Bodies? Here's What XX Studies Say." Dr. Axe, Dr. Axe, 11 Nov. 2017, draxe.com/cell-phone-health/.

"Symptoms of Children in High-Tech Classrooms" — Sinatra, Stephen T. "Re: WiFi in Schools." Received by Chairman and Trustees: Fay School, 48 Main Street, 16 July 2014, Southborough, MA.

"At the time of this writing" — Carlson, Ken. "Fourth Ripon Student Has Cancer. Parents Demand Removal of Cell Tower from School." The Modesto Bee, The Modesto Bee, 12 Mar. 2019, www.modbee. com/news/article227459649.html.

"The people of Danville, California" — Landman, Matt. 5G Denied In Danville California. YouTube, YouTube, 13 Mar. 2019, www.youtube. com/watch?v=vlnll7a58OA&feature=youtu.be.

"[A recent article] reports that Facebook" — Adams, Mike. "Facebook Bans All Content on Vaccine Awareness, Including Facts about Vaccine Ingredients, Vaccine Injury and Vaccine Industry Collusion." Natural News, 8 Mar. 2019, www.naturalnews.com/2019-03-08-facebook-bans-all-content-on-vaccine-awareness.html.

CHAPTER SIX

"Do you know what the number one cause" — Bethune, Sophie, and Angel Brownawell. "American Psychological Association Survey Shows Money Stress Weighing on Americans' Health Nationwide." American Psychological Association, American Psychological Association, 4 Feb. 2015, www.apa.org/news/press/releases/2015/02/ money-stress.

CHAPTER EIGHT

"It's 5 percent of our daily" — Kelly, Megan. "Switch on Your Brain by Dr. Caroline Leaf Dr. Caroline Leaf." Renewing All Things, 9 Feb. 2018, renewingallthings.com/spiritual-health/switch-brain-dr-caroline-leaf/.

"Did you know you can self-regulate" — "How Many Thoughts Does an Average Person Have a Day." Medical Articles RSS, 2009, www.themedicalquestions.com/psy/how-many-thoughts-does-an-average-person-have-a-day.html.

"Your brain has constant electricity" — Asprey, Dave. "How to Boost Your Alpha Brain Waves to Lower Stress and Improve Mood." Bulletproof, Bulletproof, 22 Jan. 2019, blog.bulletproof.com/alpha-brain-waves-lower-stress/.

"Russian scientists have proven visualization's" — Schmalbruch, Sarah. "Here's The Trick Olympic Athletes Use To Achieve Their Goals." Business Insider, Business Insider, 28 Jan. 2015, www.businessinsider.com/olympic-athletes-and-power-of-visualization-2015-1.

CHAPTER FOURTEEN

"Magnesium is the fourth most abundant" — "You Are Deficient in Magnesium, the Signs and How to Cure It." Get Holistic Health, 1 Jan. 2019, www.getholistichealth.com/78615/deficient-magnesium-signs-cure/?fbclid=IwAR0Z_9BZLl3UiEpAUc-0o0TtBcwtf-heVJ3_RUuHpZyOlABeHs7aQovk0ykk.

"Digestive experts agree that" — Axe, Josh. "Probiotics Benefits, Foods, Supplements & Side Effects." Dr. Axe, 15 Feb. 2019, draxe.com/probiotics-benefits-foods-supplements/.

CHRISSY HELMER

www.chrissyhelmer.com
@chrissyhelmer

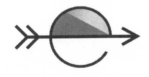

ECO CHIC

www.ecochiclife.net
@ecochiclife

1661 E Monte Vista Ave
Suite Q102
Vacaville, CA
707.624.6168
chrissy@ecochiclife.net